Tinnitus

TURNING THE VOLUME DOWN

Proven Strategies for
Quieting the Noise in Your Head

Kevin Hogan, Psy.D.

Tinnitus: Turning The Volume Down

Proven Strategies For Turning Down the Noise In Your Head

Hogan, Kevin, 1961-
Tinnitus: Turning the Volume Down, Proven Strategies for Turning
the Noise Down in Your Head
Editor: Kathy Hume Gray
Bibliography
1. Tinnitus
2. Treatment
3. Causes

ISBN:0-9709321-2-X

Cataloging In Publication Data

RF293.8.H 617.8-dc20

Published by:
Network 3000 Publishing Co.
3432 Denmark, PMB 108
Eagan, MN 55123
(612) 616-0732
Phone Toll Free: 1-888-707-1896
Fax: 952-707-1898

Printed and bound in the United States of America by:
Morris Publishing, 3212 East Highway 30, Kearney, NE 68847
1-800-650-7888

Other Books by
Kevin Hogan

Selling Yourself to Others

The Psychology of Persuasion

Talk Your Way to the Top

The Gift: A Discovery of Love, Happiness & Fulfillment

Life by Design

Through the Open Door: Secrets of Self–Hypnosis
   (with Mary Lee LaBay)

The New Hypnotherapy Handbook:
   Hypnosis and Mindbody Healing

TINNITUS: TURNING THE VOLUME DOWN

Table of Contents

CHAPTER FOUR

EVALUATING YOUR EMOTIONS & FINE TUNING
TREATMENT OPTIONS   **96**

CHAPTER FIVE

EFFECTIVE TREATMENT METHODS FOR
TINNITUS REDUCTION   **112**

Introduction

Maimonides, a philosopher, physician, scientist and rabbi who practiced medicine in the 1100s AD, treated his patients with the true art that medicine is. His advice to physicians was this:

> *It is the duty of the physician to regard the patient not as a specimen to be placed into a particular class but as an individual; to consider his constitution, his emotional state, habits, physical strength, and the immediate causes of his illness. Above all, the physician must avoid routine treatment.*

Like Kevin Hogan's, Maimonides' attitude toward medicine was not merely treatment of disease. Kevin Hogan has a positive approach to health as a definite goal worthy of determination. Kevin experienced tinnitus, and partly because of this, he treats those who suffer from it *with respect!*

He heard the usual, "You have to live with it," and he does NOT live with it. In addition he has remolded his profession to help those with tinnitus. This book is a positive example—a helping hand—a light in the darkness. Kevin once wrote a book called *The Gift: A Discovery of Love, Happiness and Fulfillment*, describing a quest for happiness. Readers discover on their quest that only by giving it (The Gift) away to everyone they meet can life be complete and whole. This book is Kevin's gift to us.

Christine Coleman, M.A., M.F.C.C.
Executive Director
Hope For Hearing Foundation
Los Angeles, California

TINNITUS: TURNING THE VOLUME DOWN

CHAPTER ONE
A Journey From Hell to Peace

Why a book about tinnitus, and, why one by me? I have written ten books but as recently as 12 years ago, I never dreamed that I would be writing a book about tinnitus treatment and therapies. 12 years ago I had never heard of the word tinnitus. Then disaster struck. I not only heard the word tinnitus, I heard the sounds at unbelievable volume day and night for 2 ½ years.

I am not an M.D., a D.O., or a psychiatrist. I am a psychotherapist. Before experiencing severely disabling tinnitus, I had aspirations significantly different from writing a tome about head noises and resolving the emotional distress of tinnitus for myself and others. I had severely disabling tinnitus from the summer of 1993 to the early winter of 1995: thirty months of hell. I worked my tinnitus into remission completely for almost one full year. Now, I occasionally experience some head noise. Perhaps once each week or month, I will lay in bed and hear that sound. It's faint, it's no longer threatening but it is a reminder to do all the right things...which I will show you.

I know exactly what you are dealing with and will leave no stone unturned in assisting you on your journey to peace. My role in your healing process is that of consultant, psychotherapist, and hypnotherapist. The best way to begin is to share with you a thumbnail sketch of my tinnitus story. After my story, we will help you prepare to write "your story" of recovery.

My Recovery from Tinnitus – and the Research I Uncovered On the Journey

August 1, 1993, 2 A.M.

The noise turned on at just over 80 dB, and I needed relief now. I knew what tinnitus was because just a few weeks before, for several hours in the night, I had experienced intense head noise that was severely loud for several hours before finally fading. I knew the noise was called tinnitus because I had looked it up in the *Encyclopedia Britannica*. I knew nothing else about it. This time, at 2 A.M., August 1, 1993, the 80+ dB noise was relentless. It woke me up out of sleep. I turned on the television and then turned the volume all the way up. I put a fan by my head on high. I couldn't stand the head noise, and the external noise failed to cover the internal noise in any significant way. I was despondent.

But I Don't Want to Take Drugs!

I called my physician as soon as his office opened. He recommended calling the American Tinnitus Association for information, and then scheduled an appointment to see me. The ATA told me there was a medication called Xanax that could reduce the noise within two to three months for most people who used it The kind old man who took my call was literally saving my life and he didn't even know it. Jack Vernon, Ph.D., gave me hope on my first day of this maddening experience. This was the beginning of my new unwanted life—life with tinnitus ringing at 70 to 80+ dB—day in and day out.

It would eventually go away, but I had no way of knowing that. I knew I had to put together a plan of action to overcome this minute–by–minute dread. After reading over a thousand abstracts, papers, and articles about tinnitus, and several serious reflective days where suicide was strategically planned, I decided that if it didn't get better soon, there was little reason to go on. Life, late that summer, was something to which I felt I could no longer meaningfully contribute.

I once used street drugs in college and learned how incredibly stupid that was. When my personal medical doctor told me Xanax may be habituating, I was torn between dealing with the drug or the noise. I didn't want to feel the "need" for a drug. I hated the idea of dependency. However, it dawned on me that if I did become dependent on a low dosage of Xanax, that would mean it was helping enough to justify the dependency. The noise was 80dB and relentless. The research was clear: 76 percent of individuals using Xanax gained relief by more than 40 percent volume reduction in their tinnitus. It would take 8 to 12 weeks for the drug to make an impact. (1)

Seventy–six percent is most people, but I was not comfortable with the odds. Never having been a lucky person, I visualized myself as part of the 24 percent who would experience no change. I started the prescription and felt groggy.

The only positive benefit in the first few days was a reduction in anxiety; there was no change in the volume. I wasn't going to just sit and wait two months for the medication to "kick in." I was still going "crazy," and I needed relief.... now!

The next step was to take some time off work and go to the library. I was finishing my doctorate in clinical hypnotherapy and working 60 hours per week. I was also spending days at home with my three–year–old daughter. A significant amount of stress was present in my life. The inter–library loan librarian was soon inundated with my requests for hundreds of articles, journals, books, periodicals, in which I was finding sanity–saving information.

We found phone numbers for the small number of specialists in the United States, and I called them. I learned that a few treatments were having success; most were not. Those treatments that were having success looked unpleasant: I read of daily injections of drugs, what I considered to be "high risk pills," surgery of the eighth nerve, and other discouraging "solutions." I became more depressed as each day passed.

The end of August was upon our small family of three, and our new motor home was sitting and waiting for me to get healthy so we could take a vacation. Driving it, though, exacerbated the three tinnitus sounds in my head. My new theory of the cause of my tinnitus was that I was having allergic reactions to something. I quit eating various foods, stayed away from electromagnetic frequencies, and decided that leaving for a vacation and a new environment might just might do the trick. At this time, I read a study in *Prevention* magazine stating that: "Sixty percent of individuals who use Seldane experience some reduction in the volume of their tinnitus." (2)

Suicide?

The study was not well done (meaning that the results might have been biased toward the medication), as far as I understood it at that time, but I decided to talk to my doctor. He agreed it was worth attempting. He knew I was on "the edge," and he wrote a script for a 30–day trial prescription. I was still taking the Xanax, and it was having no effect.

We took ten days off and drove to Cape Cod from our Minnesota home. I had taken only one vacation in the previous four years. Years before, we had visited Cape Cod and loved it; in fact, some of our fondest memories had been experienced there. From my hypnosis education I knew the psychological importance of a healing environment, so off we went to Cape Cod, my tinnitus still ringing in the high 70s.

As I sat by one of my favorite spots on the Cape, alone one day, attempting to meditate and pray, I first decided seriously that life, for me, was not worth participating in. I was seemingly useless to my wife and daughter. I felt as if the world now revolved around my noise. Everything around me was out of perspective. I was a walking bundle of nerves, depressed, with little good to say when I opened my mouth. I put a good face on for my daughter, but my wife knew that I was losing my battle and my control. I was now over thirty days into the Xanax and ten into the Seldane. All I felt was tired, groggy, and depressed.

My wife talked me out of suicide, thank God. The insurance policies would have to be put back into the safety deposit box. However, the depression and chronic fatigue continued. The noise was still incessant.

Once we were home we realized that money was running thin. School had drained savings, and our jaunt east sapped more money than we had anticipated. I had no choice but to go back to work. Ironically, I continued to help individuals in my hypnotherapy and psychotherapy practice with their various chronic illnesses. Most of my clients were improving their conditions, but I was getting nowhere. "Physician heal thyself." The phrase ran through my mind over and over.

Pamelor: Stress, Anxiety, Depression & Panic Attacks

The study had indicated that if the Seldane were to help, it would be fairly quickly. We discontinued it but continued the Xanax, knowing it could still take weeks for it to take effect. Xanax was my only hope until someone handed me a copy of the *National Enquirer* one day. *The National Enquirer*? I was desperate enough to read the article, which gave the name of a Dr. Mark Sullivan out east who had done some research on Pamelor (a tricyclic antidepressant) as a treatment for tinnitus. I remember noting that Pamelor helped about 40 percent of individuals reduce their tinnitus. (3) It was worth a try.

A simple math equation reminded me that between the Xanax,, Seldane, and Pamelor, my chances were over 95 percent that at least one would be helpful $[1-(.24x.4x.6)]$!

Pamelor also seemed to be a logical choice since I had been experiencing a significant amount of stress, anxiety, and depression for some time, even before the onset of tinnitus. The tinnitus simply made everything worse. Research I had been reading at that time clearly indicated that I was not alone. In fact, most people with tinnitus, experienced: stress (4), panic disorder (5), anxiety (6), depression (7), and/or emotional problems (8) before the onset of their tinnitus (also known as: S.P.A.D.E. or simply SPADE).

The encouraging news for me was that tinnitus, apparently, was not simply an ear phenomenon. There was a reasonable correlation between emotional distress, which is very treatable, and tinnitus, which according to most professionals, was not. In fact, the relationship between what is called subjective tinnitus and (S.P.A.D.E.) was the norm for most clients with whom I would later work.

Another interesting paper I came across noted that once an individual had tinnitus, he became far more likely to acquire other somatics (pains and illnesses) than someone without tinnitus.(9) All of this described me to a "T." How ironic, I thought.

At this point I began to believe that some form of hypnosis actually might be a useful treatment for tinnitus. Many of my clients whose illnesses and pains seemed to expand into more somatics were excellent candidates for elimination of chronic illness via hypnotherapy. I began to investigate, but my tinnitus was still in the 70+ dB range, and the hyperacusis (fear and extreme sensitivity to sound or certain sounds) I experienced was becoming more frustrating to deal with every day.

It was sometime in October when my doctor prescribed Pamelor. The tinnitus immediately skyrocketed back into the 70s and then the 80s and maybe even higher. *The tinnitus sounds moved around my head.* One very, very terrifying morning, I called the doctor and asked to be taken off the medication. He explained to me that the neurological impact the Pamelor was having in the brain, though not predictable, was reasonable, and it was still likely that it would decrease the volume. I agreed to continue, but I was scared.

Not long after that call, only a few weeks into the new prescription, *the Pamelor completely eliminated my tinnitus.* For a few days I experienced silence. It kicked in with the Xanax and for several days the tinnitus was almost completely gone. The Pamelor days would be short though, as the side effects mounted. Dry mouth, fatigue, very high blood pressure, and bloody noses were sufficient reasons for the doctor to pull the plug, saying we couldn't continue with the Pamelor. I protested, of course. I didn't care about the side effects, compared to the benefits I was receiving from the medication. Silence was wonderful, even at the price I was paying for it. I did not care if I would die in five years from hypertension or some other cause, if my head was quiet. No matter. Thanksgiving came and the Pamelor went. My medical doctor wasn't going for my argument. Zoloft, a substitute, was prescribed in its stead. The tinnitus returned, in the mid–60s range most days. The side effects were gone, except for some sexual dysfunction, but the noise had returned, albeit "quieter."

Hypnotherapy Works?!

Christmas came and went. It was a horrible holiday season. I tried to put on a happy face for friends and relatives. They had no idea what was going on inside of my head. On the "outside," in everyone else's real life world, we sold the motorcoach. I couldn't drive it, so it didn't really matter. Either the motion or the noise from driving exacerbated the tinnitus.

I was busy with clients again and my research, but I only found case studies until, early in 1994, I began uncovering reams of hypnotherapeutic research. A friend of mine, Christine Coleman, was the executive director of Hope for Hearing, at the Victor Goodhill Hearing Center, at UCLA. She also had tinnitus and helped others with tinnitus and other hearing disorders, and I asked her to work with me in finding what was "out there," that worked, in the area of treating tinnitus.

Some hypnosis research I began reading explained that:

- tinnitus needed to be treated like phantom pain with hypnotherapy. (10) (11) I had done that many times. That would actually be fairly easy, though time consuming.
- tinnitus would yield to traditional modes of regression therapy. (12)
- tinnitus could be blocked at the cortical level by hypnosis in half the cases, according to the best hypnosis experts in the world. (13)
- tinnitus could be reduced by self hypnosis tapes designed for tinnitus reduction in over 69 percent of cases if the tape program was carefully designed by the practitioner. (14)

I projected that over 80 percent of people with tinnitus should gain benefit through hypnotherapy, reducing the volume and/or the emotional impact that went along with it. I liked my chances and began practicing self hypnosis at night in lieu of the Temazepam I had been taking for sleep. It took about six weeks to really become effective at habituating to the tinnitus for sleeping, which was the worst part of my "day." At first, the self hypnosis work felt like an exercise in futility. After a month, I became proficient at it.

Occasionally, on a bad day during this habituation process, I took a Temazepam for sleep, but that was the exception and not the rule. The hypnotherapeutic tapes and self hypnosis that I created succeeded beyond my wildest dreams. I almost completely habituated the tinnitus. (Habituation means that I heard the noise but it no longer had significant meaning to me. It was annoying, not devastating...a big step.)

It was one year later. The sound was in the 40s and 50s on many days, but it rarely mattered. By 1994 year's end, the tinnitus began to permanently habituate. During all of 1995, 1996, and 1997, the tinnitus would return home and remind me that it still knew where I was, but the noise never really bothered me again. Annoying on some days to be sure, but did it trouble me? No. Sometimes the noise would come above threshold, maybe 20dB. It did not matter. I could sleep at night and not wake up to "the emergency broadcasting system." Some mornings I cried, I was so happy.

I decided it was finally time to come off the Xanax first and then the Zoloft. After a few very annoying days of letting my body readjust to being medication–free, the process was a complete success. The tinnitus did not increase after eliminating the medications. I was, in effect, cured.

Using What I Learned & Staying Current For My Clients

During 1995, my work with clients from across the country was in full stride. People from all over the world began hearing about my success through the Internet and referrals from my clients. Phone calls, faxes and emails never stopped, and they continue to this day.

And now, research released in 1995 and 1996 has validated my earlier speculations about tinnitus. In fact, the significant papers released those years were among the most important ever. They essentially prove that **various medications, tinnitus habituation training, hypnosis and other cognitive therapies like biofeedback are the most likely road to success for most individuals with tinnitus.** (The caveat is that hypnotherapy and biofeedback are practitioner dependent for success, and drugs are not. You *must* have a qualified hypnotherapist, not someone who has little or no understanding of tinnitus.)

Here are just a few of the exciting research findings that gave me hope for my clients in late 1995.

What I learned in 1995 was that tinnitus, in many sufferers, is a recursive loop of memory or, put another way, it is enmeshed into their memory and conscious awareness. This may indicate that at best, hypnosis may be able to block the tinnitus below the cortical level and from awareness, and at worst, we could teach the client to create new perceptions that would allow the conscious mind to be filled with other stimuli, and not the tinnitus. The theory and experience was validated, for me, when I read an unrelated study by Dr. Abraham Shulman, discussing where tinnitus is located in the brain. I merged his reporting about SPECT analysis (15) and my experience with hypnotherapy into a successful therapeutic regimen that continues to achieve excellent results.

I also discovered that a study of biofeedback (which is simple relaxation and manipulation of visualized images to reduce stress) proved that most people can control their emotional response to tinnitus with proper practitioner guidance. Biofeedback became popularized over 25 years ago, when it was deemed useful to measure client response to altered states of consciousness. It was discovered that most people are able to reduce their stress level through electronic monitoring. Biofeedback is generally considered to be a useful sub-field of hypnotherapy, and it is always encouraging to see positive results for tinnitus sufferers who are taught biofeedback monitored relaxation techniques.(16)

What Kind of Hypnotherapy for Tinnitus Treatment?

Hypnotherapy presents at least three different, useful models for helping people reduce the volume of their tinnitus. Although you will learn some useful information about hypnotherapy later in this book, this book is not about hypnosis. Hypnotherapy alone will not eliminate tinnitus in most people. However, an expert therapist, very familiar with tinnitus and its management, can work remarkable magic in literally "re-wiring" the brain of the tinnitus sufferer. Later in this book, I will share with you

- research that has been done in helping people turn the volume down with hypnotherapy.
- recent research about reducing volume with many other vital modalities.
- experiences of my clients and their personal successes and failures.

Finally, there is enough understanding about tinnitus and its reduction to put you on the road to a quieter life. There is not a plethora of scientific research in the tinnitus reduction field being done in 2003. Something that impacts so many gets so little attention. Nonetheless, current knowledge is sufficient to believe that if you utilize this book, you will, in all likelihood, gain significant relief from tinnitus and reduction in volume. Whether it takes you weeks, months, or a few years is an entirely different issue. It is very difficult to predict how long it will take before you experience quieter days and nights. The majority of people who follow through completely on the information in this book can expect significant improvement in as little as a few months. You will need help, though, from medical health professionals and several other people. You will need persistence and patience. You will need to make a financial investment in your healing process. You will need to make lifestyle changes. And you will be happier for your efforts.

Chapter End Notes

1. **Xanax** – The Xanax study was reported in *Arch Otolaryngology Head and Neck Surgery.* 1993:119:842–845 by R. Johnson, B. Brummett, A. Schleuning. The double blind placebo study showed 76 percent of individuals using Xanax had a volume reduction of 40 percent or more. The control group showed only 4 percent improving. Side effects were minimal and the study lasted only 12 weeks. Improvement for most began after 8 weeks on Xanax at 1.5 mg. per day total.

2. **Seldane** – study unavailable to author at press.

3. **Pamelor** – After a personal conversation with Dr. Mark Sullivan, my understanding was that he was at that time prescribing nortriptyline for tinnitus sufferers, and was

experiencing a fair degree of success. Further, results of the biofeedback study cited in number 16 below found that 27 percent of patients improved using Elavil, a close "cousin" to Pamelor.

4. **Stress** – A. Shulman in the SPECT study, noted in 15 below, states "The stress factor has been linked to cortisol accumulation resulting from a defect in its control of the hippocampus. Its accumulation has been linked to changes in mood which, over time, progress from anxiety to depression. The tinnitus patient may develop a memory not only for normal auditory stimuli but also, paradoxically, for the aberrant sound, that is tinnitus." Hundreds of studies cite excessive stress as related to tinnitus annoyance and suffering. Numerous studies cite excessive stress as highly correlated with tinnitus onset.

5. **Panic Disorder** – 56 percent of individuals with panic disorder experience tinnitus as well, according to one well done study on patients with panic disorder as the presenting symptom.

6. **Anxiety** – J. Cicocon, F. Amede, et al, in *Geriatrics,* Feb. 1995, pp. 18–25, note that "Subjective tinnitus is more common and may be due to peripheral or central auditory pathology, a metabolic abnormality, or anxiety/ depression."

7. **Depression** was reported as prevalent across the lives of 62 percent of tinnitus sufferers vs. 21 percent of a control group by Griffiths, Katon, Dobie, Sakai, Russo, in the *Journal of Psychosomatic Research.* vol. 31, no. 5. pp. 613–621, 1987. **(Current depression was reported in 48**

percent of tinnitus sufferers vs. 7 percent of the control group.)

8. **Emotional Problems** – In the same study noted in (7), the researchers noted that the number of **psychosocial problems,** and thus the resulting disability experienced, was significantly greater in the tinnitus group, compared to the controls. The authors' conclusion was that treatment needed to attend to both the tinnitus and the depression, when present. **Common challenges facing tinnitus sufferers in at least half of all cases include clinical depression (75 percent), insomnia (56 percent), adverse effects in lifestyle (93 percent), and sexual difficulties (52 percent).**

9. **Somatics** – J. Russo, W. Katon, et. al, noted in *Psychosomatics*, Vol. 6, 1994, pp. 546–56, "The results revealed that the number of lifetime medically unexplainable symptoms were significantly, independently, and positively related to increasing numbers of current and past anxiety and depressive disorders... and the worry–pessimism and impulsiveness, subscales... were positively related to the number of medically unexplained symptoms." The results suggest that somatization is associated with current and past history of psychiatric illnesses and harm avoidance in this sample of medical patients.

10. **Phantom Limb Pain** – Treatment by Dr. Milton Erickson used identical hypnotherapeutic application as his case study tinnitus client, noted in his textbook *Hypnotherapy*, with co-author Ernest Rossi, Irvington Publishing, 1979.

11. Pawel Jastreboff, in the *British Journal of Audiology*, 1993, pp. 7–17, noted that in the vast majority of cases, tinnitus is a phantom auditory perception, perceived exclusively by the patient... [and among the problems tinnitus brings] extremely strong imprinting of the tinnitus sound on the patient's central nervous system.

12. L. Ron Hubbard, *Dianetics.*: Los Angeles: Bridge Publishing, 1985.

13. Crasilneck and Hall, in *Clinical Hypnosis,* announced that 50 percent reduction in symptoms can be achieved, probably through blocking awareness at a cortical level. Supporting this theory, is the text, *Hypnosis: Current Clinical, Experimental and Forensic Practices,* edited by Michael Heap: "Hypnosis appears to be a natural choice of ... treatment for tinnitus, not only as a relaxation method but also as a means of modifying or even blocking sensory awareness." There are a number of comments and reports in the literature concerning tinnitus sufferers.

14. G. Brattberg, at the Sandvikens Hospital in Sweden did a longitudinal study of patients using a self hypnosis tape after just one session of hypnotherapy with a client. Sixty–nine percent cited improvement, regardless of cause. Three patients of the 32 studied announced a cure. Most were sleeping better, having significant improvement in critical lifestyle areas. Numerous other studies support Brattberg's findings.

15. A. Shulman, A. Strashun, et al. discussed at the Triological Society, 1993, NY, that "SPECT results of brain demonstrate for the first time the in vivo significance of the organacity of brain for a central type tinnitus... Auditory

function can be considered to involve multiple neural networks reflecting various attributes of hearing... It can be speculated that a short term memory is established for tinnitus in the medial temporal lobe memory system which becomes stored in associated areas of the neo–cortex. A paradoxical memory for tinnitus may cause the tinnitus to become clinically manifest as a severely disabling tinnitus."

16 L. Podoshin, Y. Ben-David, et. al., researched the differences of tinnitus in both resting and active situations for their patients. **43.5 percent of biofeedback patients experienced improvement at rest and 24 percent during activity, outperforming those using the drug Elavil.**

Key Points to Remember in this Chapter

- You don't have to completely understand how tinnitus works to experience quieter days and peace of mind.
- My personal experience has been duplicated by numerous other people. Be patient and allow yourself to remain optimistic.
- If one method of treatment or therapy fails, there is still nothing to worry about. It may take several treatments and several months, before you notice significant changes in your tinnitus.
- I was an emotional wreck through much of my tinnitus experience and I still made it through. You can too.
- Most medical and mental health practitioners know very little about tinnitus. It will be your job to learn what they need to know to help you.
- There is no shame and much benefit to be gained by utilizing medications such as anti-depressants and anti-anxiety medications for tinnitus reduction.
- Complementary therapies such as hypnosis and biofeedback can be very helpful, but you must have a skilled and empathetic practitioner to help you.

CHAPTER TWO
Tinnitus:
Understanding the Noise

Until a person has experienced tinnitus, there is no way to explain the distress and frustration you experience. It is possible to reproduce the noise of your tinnitus for someone on a synthesizer, or possibly in an audiologist's office. You could turn up the volume, match the pitch of your tinnitus, and let someone listen to it. There is, however, something very different about listening to a distressing sound for a few moments, knowing that in seconds it will be turned off, and living with a disturbing noise that you think will never quiet. Suffering from tinnitus goes beyond distress for many. The noise sometimes can be maddening, and many people have committed suicide because of it.

Two unrelated people experiencing severe tinnitus in 1997 became clients of mine after each watched a sibling (brothers in both instances) take his own life because of tinnitus. At this time there is no reason to believe that severe tinnitus is genetic, but one thing is certain: Very few experiences in human life are as intensely devastating as suffering from severe tinnitus. This book is written for the person who is suffering from tinnitus.

Tinnitus, according to tinnitus expert, Dr. Abraham Shulman, can be defined as, "a disorder of auditory perception due to an altered state of excitation/inhibition in neuronal networks resulting in a dysynchrony of neuronal signaling. The underlying mechanism is that dysynchronization, that is, a lack of synchrony or interference in timing of the discharge rate and phase locking of the auditory signal having a location peripheral, central or both" (*International Tinnitus Journal*, Shulman, 1995).

In lay language, I might define tinnitus as **any noise produced in either the ear and/or the unconscious portions of the brain that is experienced, in large part, from the conscious portion of the mind spending time in a feedback loop that is constantly moving from hearing noise to experiencing negative emotions, ad infinitum.**

In simpler terms yet, *tinnitus is noise, heard in the head or the ear, that is generated from within the individual.* Severe tinnitus is that which causes the individual distress in the form of anxiety, depression, stress, panic, emotional and/or communication problems.

How Does My Tinnitus Compare to Others?

Millions and millions of people all across the world suffer from tinnitus. The American Tinnitus Association reports that in the U.S., an estimated 12 million people have tinnitus to a disturbing degree. There is no objective method of measuring how "bad" someone has it; however, there is one classification system that I find particularly useful as a scale for understanding the distress caused by tinnitus.

I have made a few minor adaptations to a system developed by A. Glorig for you to evaluate your tinnitus. Circle the best answer to each of the following questions, then tally the circled points and compare your total with the rating at the bottom of the survey.

---

1. Is the noise... ?

Constant	3
Intermittent, more on than off	2
Intermittent, more off than on	1

2. Does it prevent you from going to sleep... ?

Yes, frequently	2
Yes, infrequently	1
No	0

3. Is it worse in the quiet?

Yes	1
No	2

4. Is it worse when you are not busy doing something?

Yes	1
No	2

5. What does it sound like?

High pitched tone	2
Low pitched tone	2
Rushing air	1
Static	2
Other	1

6. How much does it bother you?

	Mildly	1
	Moderately	2
	Severely	3
YOUR TOTAL		

The California Scale

Slight 5
Mild 6/7
Mild to Moderate 8/9
Moderate...10/11
Severe ....12+

Why is this Noise in My Head?!

Many people have asked whether their tinnitus is some kind of a curse from God or a hallucination caused by the devil. I can assure you that it is neither. Tinnitus is as real as anything else you can see or hear. It does exist. It is not imaginary.

Have you ever looked at the clear sky and seen "floaters"? Floaters are normally nothing to be concerned with, but at times they can be annoying. They are often caused by fragmenting of cells in the eye that are registering in the retina. Similarly, tinnitus is often caused by just a little damage in something called the **cochlea**. The cochlea is part of the inner ear that is critical to our hearing external sounds. If you ever look at a diagram of the middle and inner ear, the cochlea is the part that looks like a snail shell. Inside the shell are tiny sensory cells (hair cells) that respond to sound and send nerve signals to the brain. Damage to these hair cells can and often does, cause tinnitus.

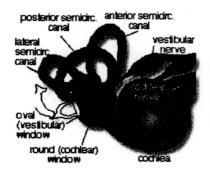

posterior semicirc. canal
anterior semicirc. canal
lateral semicirc canal
vestibular nerve
oval (vestibular) window
round (cochlear) window
cochlea

In many individuals, tinnitus can be likened to phantom limb pain. It is important to understand precisely what is meant by this. Phantom limb pain hurts as much as any pain you will ever experience. Pain is a signal from somewhere in the body to the brain that tells the brain that something is wrong. However, in reality, there is no need for phantom limb pain since there is no present–time physical cause for it. An example will help make this clear.

In my session work, many war veterans have reported pain in a "leg" or an "arm" that was either removed or destroyed in combat. When this happens, one part of the brain is telling another part of the brain that there is pain where the limb once was. How is this possible? There are a few explanations. One is that there is cellular memory, and that each cell has its own piece of memory. Each cell in our body communicates with other cells in our body. Interestingly, these components in the body do not always tell the brain important bits of information, such as the fact that the limb is no longer there and pain is not necessary! The brain only remembers how painful the leg was, and this is the last bit of memory about the leg it has. It repeats the memory like a cybernetic loop, and continues to do so until it is told, normally in hypnotherapy, that it can stop.

33

The cessation of pain in phantom limb–experiencing patients is normally time consuming, but not "difficult." Hypnotherapy is remarkably effective in the healing process, as will be discussed later in this book. A key to success is returning the client in his mind to the incident of the trauma, and bringing this repressed, unconscious memory into conscious awareness. This "connection" and re-association normally reduces or entirely eliminates the pain. In both phantom limb pain and tinnitus, hypnotherapy is not the only solution available. In just a few pages you will read about how one case of phantom limb pain was eliminated without hypnotherapy, as a model for how you can reduce your tinnitus volume and distress.

> It repeats the memory like a cybernetic loop, and continues to do so until it is told, normally in hypnotherapy, that it can stop.

Tinnitus, of course, has dozens of potential causes. Those causes that we can easily discover and, hopefully, correct, are called "pathological." **Pathological** means we can find a pathology, or cause, processes, and development. The largest number of people with severe tinnitus experience what is known as **"subjective idiopathic tinnitus."** Subjective means that only you can hear the noise. Idiopathic means that the pathology is unknown, and we know what tinnitus means.

This book is written for you, the tinnitus sufferer, and your medical and mental health professional, to assist you in the process of healing after all standard diagnostics and treatments have been exhausted.

Your medical doctor may be unaware of the vast number of pathologies for tinnitus. The following outline will be of some usefulness for your doctor. Feel free to share it with him or her. This outline is based upon the classifications of tinnitus by Ross Coles, MRC Institute of Hearing Research in Nottingham, England (1995). It will present you and your doctor with some, but not all classifications of tinnitus. It should be noted that *there may be multiple classifications of tinnitus for any one individual. In one instance, tinnitus may have two or more causes. In another instance, tinnitus sounds heard may include several different and distinct sounds with different causes.*

Classification of Tinnitus:

By Type and Site of Underlying Disorder

I. Physiological

    A. Muscular (hums)

    B. Vascular

    C. Brownian

II. Spontaneous Otoacoustic Emissions

III. Temporary Dysfunction

    A. Noise induced

    B. Drug induced

    C. Toxemic

IV. Pathological

    A. Extra–auditory

        1. Muscular

        2. Respiratory

        3. Vascular

    B. Conductive

        1. Enhancement

            a. Coincident

b. Consequent of Meniere's

c. Other

2. Movements

a) External Ear

b) Middle Ear

C. Sensorineural

1. Sensory

2. Peripheral neural

3. Central Neural

D. Associated

1. Cervical

2. Temporomandibular

E. Psychological

1. Hallucinatory

2. Imagery

V. Pseudo–Tinnitus

A. Environmental

B. Feigned

Tinnitus, as clearly noted in the outline above, is not experienced solely because of hearing loss. In fact, tinnitus is not experienced because of any specific disease or malfunction. The noise heard in your head is very real, whether or not you have hearing loss. The cause is often largely irrelevant when it comes to the therapeutic interventions you will undertake. The deaf who have tinnitus make up a small minority of the people who suffer from tinnitus. This book offers the deaf person with severe tinnitus strategies for improvement as well. The fact that a person is deaf does not mean she or he is more likely to have severe tinnitus than anyone else. For the deaf person, severe tinnitus is often more distressing, simply because there is no external sound to interfere with the tinnitus.

What You Can Expect From This Book

This book will help eliminate the term "subjective idiopathic tinnitus" from the mouths of all those interested in the field of tinnitology. After reading this book you will realize that your tinnitus is not "invisible." Your tinnitus is emanating from a very specific place in the brain (and/or possibly the ear), and with the information in this book, you will be able to help your medical professionals help you improve your life situation.

What you should know now is that there is hope for quieter and better days ahead. There is more than hope. Increasing numbers of people are experiencing remission from tinnitus — experiencing volume reduction and less distress. There is every reason to believe you will be among that number very soon.

Several effective treatments and therapies for tinnitus reduction are scientifically proven to be safe. Some of the drug treatments (sometimes referred to as pharmacological in this book) have side effects. Most of the therapies you will read about have no side effects at all. This book will clearly show you that almost all persons with tinnitus can reduce the volume of the noise they are hearing in their head and gain relief from the distress associated with the noise. There is one catch. The number of medical and mental health practitioners in the health care community aware of what tinnitus really is and how to treat it is very small. This book will help you make your health care professionals aware of the most recent research and studies available in treating your tinnitus.

This book is your road map, but *you* have to drive the car. There is a great deal to learn and evaluate before you begin "treating" your tinnitus. This book is intended to show you all of the major roads to a more peaceful life. It will not solve all of your problems. Simply turning the pages of this book will not make the tinnitus go away. In fact, reading about tinnitus may actually increase the volume, simply because the brain is focusing on the word, sensation, and experience! This book will show you how to develop a team of professionals to help you on your quest. It will outline exactly what you will need each doctor, osteopath, audiologist, hypnotherapist, and others to do to help you. Finally, you should know that this book is based on dozens of scientific studies, my experience in helping others reduce the volume of their tinnitus, and my own road to peace.

> What you should know now is that there is hope for quieter and better days ahead.

You will find some of my own speculative thought in the pages of this book. Tinnitus research is not complete and we will know even more in ten years than we do today. What works for most people is not guaranteed to work for everyone. For example: A medication that eliminates a problem for one person can have no significant effect with another person. A medication that eliminates a problem for me may have side effects that make the medication less appealing for someone else.

No one needs to tell you that tinnitus volume, and even frequency, can vary from day to day and even hour to hour inside your head. In some people, the sound can move from one side of the head to the other. Many respected medical doctors tell patients with tinnitus "Learn to live with it," and "Nothing I can do." They are mistaken on both counts. The medical doctor can do a great deal for you. You may or may not eventually be completely rid of the noise; many people will be. This book, for the first time tells you what "subjective idiopathic tinnitus" is, its origins, and exactly what can be done for relief. It is written in lay English (with a few exceptions where scientific discussion is necessary, so that you can share the information with your medical and mental health practitioners), but that doesn't mean that some sections will not be difficult to understand. You are about to learn information of which most medical doctors are unaware. It will be your job, as the person suffering from tinnitus, to share this information with your physician, in a careful, responsible, and methodical manner.

If you utilize the information in this book to your maximum ability, you will, in all likelihood, experience significantly quieter tinnitus volumes in less than two years. Some people will experience significant improvement in a matter of weeks after beginning treatment or therapies based upon the information in this book. For some people, the tinnitus will literally disappear and, even if yours does not, you almost certainly will not be as distressed by this maddening disorder as you are today.

What is this Noise in My Head?

The ringing hasn't seemed to want to stop. For some reason it might sound like roaring or buzzing or sizzling. Some people hear crickets or sizzling. All of these kinds of sound are emanating from inside the brain or the ear (or both) and for many, these sounds can be debilitating. Whatever it is that you hear, it is more than annoying. These sounds are called *tinnitus*.

Tinnitus was once thought to be only an "ear" problem, and it was believed that everyone heard tinnitus in the ear. This is not correct. In approximately 50 percent of cases where an tinnitus sufferer had the **auditory nerve** cut (the auditory nerve leads from the ear to the brain), the person's tinnitus continued with little or no change. The horror of this situation was that the patient was now deaf in the ear after the nerve was cut. What these tragic surgeries demonstrated is positive proof that tinnitus is often generated within the brain. Thankfully, in the 1990s and beyond, surgeries to cut the auditory nerve for the purpose of eliminating tinnitus are rare.

In 96 percent of cases, tinnitus can be heard only by the person whose head it is in. The medical term for this is **subjective tinnitus.** Objective tinnitus is contrasted to subjective tinnitus in that it can be heard by another person, usually with a stethoscope. This program was designed for the person who suffers from subjective tinnitus, but it will aid the person with objective tinnitus as well. You are, no doubt, somewhat anxious about these noises. You may be frustrated that few people, if any, have useful ideas for you about reducing or eliminating the noise and, maybe more importantly, the emotional distress that accompanies this noise. If this is true, you can rest assured that you are "normal." Experiencing a noise that doesn't stop is enough to make just about anyone a little on edge. Millions of people in the United States **suffer** from tinnitus. However, you will be interested to know that *most people who have tinnitus do not suffer from* *tinnitus*. For them, it is simply "there." In this book you will learn how to stop suffering from tinnitus.

Some people develop tinnitus because they smoke, drink alcohol, or use simple antibiotics or pain killers that can cause tinnitus. Frequently, the cessation of the offending substance will be enough to eliminate the noise completely. Although this is true in less than 5 percent of cases I have worked with, it is always a nice, quick end to an annoying problem.

> Experiencing a noise that doesn't stop is enough to make just about anyone a little on edge.

"Tinnitus is a symptom," is what "they" say, but sometimes they are wrong. Tinnitus *can be* a symptom. It can also be little more than a very loud and emotionally distressing "memory loop. Tinnitus can be the only presenting difficulty in some people. It can be the only "physical" symptom of emotional problems such as anxiety, depression, or severe stress. It can also be a sign of anemia or diabetes. It can be a signal of a tumor that needs to be removed. It can be a signal generated from the inner or middle ear. It can be a symptom of otosclerosis. Tinnitus can be, but is not necessarily, related to inner ear disorders. In some people, the middle or inner ear is the culprit in locating the sound generator of tinnitus. This book will also show that some people experience tinnitus because of immense pressure on the eighth nerve and/or the surrounding cranial areas including the TMJ. An equal or larger number of people have no tinnitus being generated in their middle or inner ear. For them it sounds off from a key area for memory in the brain that we will discuss in some detail later.

In the past decade, research that can dramatically reduce or eliminate your tinnitus has been taking place, but far too quietly. The conventional "wisdom" that said, "You are just going to have to learn to live with it," really didn't help much. You *may* have to do just that, but if you do, this book will show you *how*.

Have you been under a great deal of stress? Have you experienced depression? One goal of this book is to show you how to eliminate the negative emotions related to tinnitus. These emotions are often manifested in depression, stress, anxiety, panic disorder, and emotional illnesses. You will need to take an active role in pursuing proper medical support in your quest for peace. Tinnitus reduction is not a passive process.

The Company You Keep

When tinnitus first onsets, the person normally feels that they are the only one that has tinnitus. This is simply not true. William Shatner (Star Trek), Barbara Streisand (The Way We Were), Peter Townsend (The Who), Tony Randall (The Odd Couple), David Letterman, and former President Reagan are all tinnitus sufferers who probably felt the same way. Knowing this does not make the tinnitus you have any quieter, but it does temporarily keep you in good company until that time!

The Oregon Health Sciences University has published on the Internet important demographic and experiential information about people who suffer from tinnitus. Here are a few of the little known facts they have made public from their own data base research. (Note: This is my personal interpretation of their data, which was recently made public. For more information, contact OHSU.)

■ 51 percent of individuals with tinnitus became aware of their tinnitus in a gradual fashion. The tinnitus started out slowly and gradually persisted.

■ 7 percent of individuals had a rapid onset of tinnitus: Their tinnitus onset in a time span of 1 to 4 weeks.

■ 39 percent of individuals reported their tinnitus came on suddenly, in less than 1 week.

Another interesting area of research the OHSU reported was what, if anything, people associated with the onset of their tinnitus (illnesses, accidents, special circumstances, etc.). By far the most common answer, 42 percent, was that the tinnitus sufferer did not know anything that was related to the onset. Forty–two percent of all tinnitus listeners have no idea what was even partially responsible for the onset of tinnitus. When medical practitioners are unable to determine the cause of tinnitus it is called **idiopathic.**

The OHSU data base research also revealed the following:

■ 13 percent of individuals reported long durations of noise as a precipitating circumstance to their tinnitus.

■ 16 percent reported head or neck injury as a precipitating circumstance.

■ 4 percent reported a brief noise was a precipitating circumstance.

■ 7 percent reported that an explosion like gunfire or fireworks was a precipitating cause.

■ 23 percent reported that medical conditions or treatments for medical conditions accounted for the individual's onset. These included ear infections, ear problems, sinus problems, medications and drugs, and other illnesses.

■ 42 percent or more of those participating in the research had no key to the mystery they were attempting to solve.

Tinnitus has also been found to present itself in several fashions. First, noises occur at different frequencies. Second, they occur at different levels of volume. Third, are the *number of noises heard.*

■ 53 percent of tinnitus sufferers reported hearing one noise.

■ 26 percent reported two different noises.

■ 10 percent reported three noises.

■ 6 percent reported more than three noises.

Once an individual has experienced the onset of persistent tinnitus, only 2 percent of listeners hear their tinnitus less than when first experiencing tinnitus. This means that the vast majority of all sufferers have a great deal of their attention focused on the noises. The impact of tinnitus on the individual is powerful. With only 2 percent noticing their tinnitus less, it is obvious that there is a dramatic need to learn to put our conscious attention elsewhere.

Another very important element of tinnitus is that the location from where it is being heard can change. Eleven percent of people report that their tinnitus has changed locations by moving from one side **(unilateral)**, to both sides **(bilateral)**. Another 2 percent report significant change in locations.

Sleeplessness is a very important presenting problem among tinnitus listeners. When asked if tinnitus interferes with their sleep, participants answered:

No	29 percent
Sometimes	44 percent
Yes. Often	25 percent

One of the key goals of this book is to lead you to inexpensive tools that are perfectly safe for falling asleep as peacefully as possible.

Tinnitus also causes its listeners to suffer in yet another way. When asked the question, Do you feel tinnitus has caused you significant problems in **irritability or nervousness?** respondents answered as follows:

No	18 percent
Sometimes	42 percent
Yes	38 percent

You can contact a local hypnotherapist to create an audio tape for sleep disorders. Most charge less than $200 for such a service. The Tinnitus Reduction Program audio cassette program, mentioned previously, contains a hypnotherapy audiocassette that has the specific goal of reducing the emotional impact of tinnitus. You will find this a valuable tool. Once you know, at the conscious level, that tinnitus is not a life threatening problem, it becomes something over which you can gain a great deal of control at the unconscious (amygdala) level.

Will the Noise Go Away?

It very well might. A set of figures from a Chicago hospital recently revealed that about 25 percent of tinnitus listeners will one day notice their tinnitus just disappears. In nearly 50 percent, the tinnitus listener will notice a reduction in volume, and the other quarter will be served by therapeutic intervention. That makes the odds swing in your favor quite a bit, doesn't it? When you consider that this hospital did not have all the information you now have, your odds go up again.

Helping Others On the Road

A few pages back, you read about what happened to me when I was suffering from tinnitus. Before we go on to helping you understand your tinnitus and gain relief, this is a good time to share with you some specifics about my experience in working with other suffering people, just like you and me.

Since early 1995 (as I write this in February of 2003), I have worked with over 1000 clients suffering from severe tinnitus. Some of these people had been turned away by many health professionals with whom they had pleaded for help. Many of my clients have been to this country's leading experts (whose research is highlighted in the pages to follow). Almost 30 people I have seen in the past few years spent nearly $100,000 in search of the answers that would lead them to peace of mind and quieter tinnitus.

I was able to help most of them. A few did not experience significant improvement, and for them my heart breaks. Having had tinnitus and suffered greatly from it, I want everyone to achieve dramatic improvement. I can report that almost everyone can improve dramatically.

My experience with tinnitus sufferers goes beyond 1000 clinical clients with tinnitus, averaging 18 session hours per client. I have personally corresponded and talked at length with more than 5,000 more wonderful people who suffer distress from tinnitus. I have given consultations by mail, phone, and email during the same eight–year span.

Today, in 2003, it is becoming increasingly difficult to help everyone who has questions and needs help now. I wish I had all the answers to all of the problems that are presented to me. No one does have all the answers because the diagnostic equipment for tinnitus is simply not available to the everyday medical or mental health practitioner.

Like any professional, I must refer some of my clients who need additional assistance to other experts including, but not limited to the offices and related professional teams and associations of Jack Vernon (Portland, OR), Abraham Shulman (New York, NY), Pawel Jastreboff (Baltimore), Stephen Nagler (Atlanta), John House (Los Angeles), Ross Coles, Jonathon Hazell, Aage Moller, Denk, Felix and Ehrenberger (all in Europe), and finally, Kitahara (Japan). There are other professionals in the United States and around the world, but these are the key researchers whose work has drawn my attention as being on track and likely to succeed with their patients.

If I have neglected a full time tinnitus professional, please contact the publisher and we will consider inclusion in our 2007 edition of this book.

Medical and mental health professionals who use and recommend a multi-modal approach in working with patients tend to succeed with greater regularity than those who use their "pet modality." Here in Minnesota, we normally succeed in reducing volume and distress in the long term for most people. There is not just one modality for reducing tinnitus volume. In fact there isn't even a "best" method. We are just now beginning to experience with clients what was once thought impossible: tinnitus remission. We do not know how long remissions will last and can only speculate as to the likelihood of long term prognosis for those who experience silence after severe tinnitus.

There are numerous excellent modalities of help for you to pursue. It will be, in large part, up to you which paths you will follow for your own healing process. In the United States, only a handful of clinics and practitioners are assisting people who suffer from tinnitus on a full time basis. Of those who are, many are making fine progress. Progress is being made in other parts of the world as well.

Scientific research in neural activity of both the brain and ear is confirming the real life experience of thousands with tinnitus and hundreds of people who are improving their situation. The brain is a complex organ. As progress is made in understanding it, concurrent progress is occurring in understanding tinnitus.

We now know that tinnitus is not just an "ear problem" or "hearing disorder." Sometimes suffering from tinnitus has nothing to do with the ear in any significant way. It always (yes, always) has something to do with the brain. We can guess with some level of accuracy as to the cause of any one individual's tinnitus. However, even with audiograms, MRIs, blood work, and psychological case analysis, we are only relatively certain (about 70 percent) in each person's case as to the specific mechanism of tinnitus generation. What appears to be certain cochlear synaptic tinnitus often is not. (Or it may be, and it did not matter in treating it as such.) What seems to be neurological (within the brain) in generation sometimes turns out to be tinnitus generated from the person's cochlea.

There are few absolutes in diagnosing, treating, and performing therapy with those afflicted with this noisy menace. As you turn the following pages, you are going to learn how to make your own best guess as to the origin of your tinnitus. You will learn the best current therapies and treatments for severe tinnitus. You will learn whom to call. Be prepared, though, for the very short list of experienced professionals who regularly work with people presenting severe tinnitus. The list is very, very small.

Remember that the noises being listened to are heard, in all cases, from within the brain, and for some the generator is the inner ear. In many cases, both the ear and brain "cooperate" in generating the sound you call tinnitus. For most tinnitus sufferers, all attempts at escaping the noise have been futile. The medical establishment continues to shrug its collective shoulders. Little do they realize, they have many answers for you. That is why I strongly encourage you to take this book to your medical practitioner. If that practitioner is truly interested in helping you, he or she will now be able to set you on the road to recovery. Many myths about tinnitus will soon fall by the wayside. This book will point out errors in traditional treatment of tinnitus and hyperacusis, and their management. You will learn what works and what is nothing short of voodoo.

Volume reduction will be achieved by most, and for a significantly smaller number, remission (undetermined periodic elimination) is a very realistic objective. For all people who suffer from tinnitus, *tinnitus needs to be carefully and thoroughly understood, and carefully diagnosed by a licensed medical practitioner before beginning any therapy or treatment.* A medical practitioner who is ignorant of tinnitus reduction strategies is not stupid. Ignorance is lack of awareness. The medical practitioner never had access to this information in medical school. Seek the help of a practitioner who wants to go the extra mile to help you.

Tinnitus is noise that, in some cases, begins as

> Seek the help of a practitioner who wants to go the extra mile to help you.

the result of a middle or inner ear disorder. Later it may become thoroughly enmeshed in the neurology of the brain and literally become a "persistent looping memory." You will begin to understand how tinnitus persists long after the original stimulus for the tinnitus is gone, as you read on.

Once you understand how tinnitus is often generated, you will learn how to "re-wire your brain" to reduce the volume of tinnitus. Some people will succeed with the tools mentioned in this book, without pursuing additional assistance. This group will be in the minority. Most people will need to seek help from competent medical practitioners, osteopaths, and very adept and experienced psychotherapists and hypnotherapists. Later, we will discuss how to select a medical practitioner and a hypnotherapist. You probably will have to do some traveling if this book's contents don't meet your long term goals. Some will come here to Minnesota. Others will go to the University of Maryland, Atlanta, Oregon, or Los Angeles. Some will go to New York. Europe may end up on your itinerary. Or, you may be able to get the help you need in your own hometown.

Regardless of the treatments you select, you must realize that tinnitus reduction is a long–term process. In order to understand how tinnitus can be quieted, let us begin by considering the ways other sensory errors or phantom perceptions that others experience happen. I want you to look at how people experience these seemingly unusual experiences, and then consider how they can then overcome sensory "errors." We will use phantom limb pain as a useful analogy for tinnitus, and our starting point in Chapter Three.

Key Points to Remember in This Chapter

- There are many different kinds and causes of tinnitus.
- Have your medical doctor refer you to a specialist so you can have a CT Scan or MRI to rule out a tumor. While rare, they do occur.
- Your emotional state of mind is inextricably linked to the distress you experience from your tinnitus.
- Have blood tests done to determine if you have any deficiencies, including Zinc and Magnesium. Also, have your doctor determine if you are hyperinsulinemic or diabetic.
- Most people with tinnitus experience problems sleeping. Ask your medical doctor for help.
- Most people with tinnitus are irritable because of the tinnitus. Communicate effectively with those around you so they understand what you are experiencing.
- Half of all people with tinnitus hear more than one sound of tinnitus in their head (ears).
- Some of the most successful people in the world have tinnitus. You are by no means alone.

CHAPTER THREE
Your Tinnitus Address – Helping It Find a New Home

A Metaphor for Tinnitus:
Very Real "Phantom Perception"

Have you ever heard stories of the veterans of wars whose pain–ridden limbs were amputated, due to irreversible infections and damage? Many still felt pain in their "limbs" long after the limbs were physically removed. The phenomenon became known as phantom limb pain, although there was nothing phantom about it. The pain was excruciatingly real. Part of the brain was unaware of the limb's eradication and the pain continued. For 50 years hypnotherapists have had success in reducing or eliminating phantom pain. Meanwhile, medical science remained stumped, ignoring the obvious evidence that such pain was successfully being removed through hypnosis. How could hypnotherapy be successful, and medical science miss the boat?

For the answer to this question we turn to current research and understanding in neuroscience.

When brain cells lose an "old job," they find a "new job." Research by Nobel Prize Winners, Torsten Weisel and David Hubel at Harvard Medical School has proved this notion beyond a reasonable doubt. Weisel and Hubel have have done no research into tinnitus of which I am aware, and would probably be conservative in commenting on tinnitus, if asked. Nevertheless, their research into the way the brain stores sensory data is critical to tinnitus reduction.

Certain impulse–conducting cell (neuronal) connections in the brain create and "remember" the perception of sound. When a sound that was once experienced is no longer there, in this case of hearing loss for example, the cells have nothing to do. The cells apparently find a new job. If they can no longer perceive and interpret sounds, at least they can go and get a new job helping to generate sound for the brain. The cells and the interconnections are unaware that this looping memory is unwanted by the individual. They are simply "doing their job."

A related experience is described in Pulitzer Prize Winner Ronald Kotulak's *Inside the Brain,* published by Andrews McMeel in 1997.

> *Those notions [of severed nerves generating pain]*
> *began to crumble with the results from experiments*
> *on monkeys. When one finger was immobilized, brain*
> *cells controlling the useless finger switched their*
> *allegiance to brain cells that control other parts of*
> *the hand. The process of reallocating duties from one*
> *part of the brain to another is possible because of the*
> *brain's great plasticity. It is now understood to be the*

*reason stroke patients can regain speech and other
functions through rehabilitation.*

In the case noted above, the brain worked for the good of
the monkeys and patients, respectively.

What happens when the brain acts on its own, to the
detriment of the individual, by creating phantom limb pain or
something like tinnitus? Kotulak discusses this in his book. He
describes the case of "Derrick," who later worked with Dr.
Vilaynur Ramchandran at UC San Diego. Derrick's arm was
amputated after a motorcycle accident. Derrick began
experiencing phantom limb paralysis and pain. (His brain cells
got new jobs.) Eight years after the amputation, Derrick agreed
to participate in a series of experiments with Dr.
Ramchandran—experiments, it was hoped, that would reduce
or eliminate the phantom limb pain Derrick had experienced
for eight years.

*With Derrick's eyes closed, Ramchandran touched
his cheek and asked where he felt sensation. Derrick
said it felt like his phantom hand had been touched.
Then Ramchandran brushed a cotton swab across
Derrick's jaw. This time he said he felt movement
across his missing arm.*

*Since the areas in the brain that regulate the arms
and face are adjacent, brain cells that had controlled
the missing limb crossed over to the area controlling
the face. Brain wave studies confirmed the rewiring
had taken place.* (The old cells took new jobs.)

*But despite this crossover, that part of the brain
could not totally give up its former control of the
paralyzed missing limb. Those brain cells insisted*

that the missing limb was *still there.* **The brain cells continued to send messages around a useless closed loop, a painful reminder of their past duties.**

Derrick eventually broke the painful spell by learning how to disconnect the faulty wiring in his brain. He did it with the help of a long narrow box built by Ramchandran.

A mirror inside ran the length of the box. When Derrick put his remaining arm in the box, the mirror made it appear to Derrick's brain that there were two arms in the box! Derrick told himself that when he would lift a bucket or do other exercises, he was doing it with both arms. (In hypnosis, this is called a positive hallucination; it can be very useful in some therapeutic contexts.)

Derrick tricked his brain into thinking that he had two arms. After eight years, the phantom limb now "experienced" sensation, and no more pain. He had succeeded in correcting the flawed wiring in his brain. **Derrick literally re-wired his brain, and this is our goal for people who suffer from tinnitus.** Using a multi-modal approach to treating tinnitus, we should be able to successfully re-wire most people's brains, given time and very skilled therapists. Primarily, this process will include Tinnitus Habituation Therapy, specific medications, and three specific and distinct hypnotherapeutic procedures. Other treatments and therapies will be important, but play a more or less minor role. These will also be discussed in great detail later.

Is It All in the Ear?

Long after Van Gogh cut off his ear, his tinnitus continued. Long after thousands of people opted to have surgeons cut their auditory nerve, their tinnitus persisted and grew louder. In fact, *half of all patients having the eighth nerve (the auditory nerve) cut still have tinnitus.* How could this possibly be if tinnitus is in the ear? The answer, of course, is that tinnitus is only generated "in the ear" in about half of the cases, and even then, that is only a single component of a much greater auditory–brain phenomenon.

> Tinnitus research is revealing more and more that tinnitus suffering is an "emotional brain" phenomenon.

For nearly a century, the tinnitus sufferer has asked the ENT (Ear, Nose, & Throat doctor) to solve the problem of tinnitus. For a century, the tinnitus sufferer has regularly sought help from the wrong person. There are definite instances when tinnitus is caused by any number of difficulties in the middle or inner ear. The leading physical cause of tinnitus appears to be exposure to loud noise. However, even with exposure to loud noise, we now know that tinnitus is not predictable simply from sound exposure, short term or long. Other variables are involved in the tinnitus equation. Even more variables are involved in the equation of predicting who will suffer from tinnitus and who will simply experience the noise in an irrelevant fashion. These variables are uncovered in the client's history and emotional variables. The skilled and experienced practitioner of hypnosis has a great advantage in assisting the tinnitus sufferer's healing process.

Tinnitus research is revealing more and more that **tinnitus suffering is an "emotional brain" phenomenon.** This fact adds greater certainty that we can begin to focus on solutions that can meet the challenge. The solution involves re-wiring the brain. More specifically, we are going to slow down activity on neural pathways that are tinnitus creators, and we are going to create new neural pathways where tinnitus does not exist. As in Derrick's case, this will take time; it will sometimes test your patience; and it will be worth your time and effort.

Your brain is an incredible creation. Among its many important functions, it is the storehouse of your memories and experiences. It is in the brain that we hear, and it is in the brain that we remember sound. Although the ear acts as a sensory perceiving organ, it does not actually "hear" anything. The ear is the conduit of soundwaves and the magical transformer of sound waves into electrical impulses that shoot into the brain at blazing speed. The ear is where the body is balanced and equilibrium controlled, in large part. However, the ear doesn't hear anything.

> We are going to slow down activity on neural pathways that are tinnitus creators, and we are going to create new neural pathways where tinnitus does not exist.

Recall the voice of someone you love. Unless you were deaf from birth you were easily able to do this, weren't you? Even if you were profoundly deaf today, the voice of a loved one is normally an easy memory to access with conscious recall.

Long after people become deaf, they continue to hear sounds in their dreams. When you feel a certain way or have certain important decisions to make, you may hear the voice of a deceased parent or friend or your own voice, in your head. Some people, of course, hear these voices all day long, to the point that it becomes a problem. The brain, in all these cases, is working very hard, but needs re-wiring in some fashion.

The implications for those people who listen to tinnitus are profound. Like anything else in the brain, tinnitus can be altered through pharmacological means, or by altering states of consciousness in natural ways, including but not limited to hypnosis and visualization, and to a lesser degree, meditation, yoga, biofeedback, NLP, and other consciousness–altering technologies.

If you are able to achieve complete remission of tinnitus, it is still likely that you will be able to remember (experience) and bring the noise(s) to conscious awareness long after your tinnitus volume has "disappeared." Memories can fade, but like the voice of the loved one, the memory is there. It can be accessed mistakenly or intentionally. As you hear your tinnitus, realize that you are not doing anything "wrong." Your conscious awareness is simply traveling highways that have tinnitus taking up space on the road.

When considering your goals with tinnitus reduction you may want to subdivide your healing goals into two areas.

1. Reduce the volume level.
2. Reduce the level of suffering.

Therefore, we are looking for at least two solutions to at least two problems. One is to reduce the loudness of the noise and the other is to reduce the distress of the individual. Sometimes, achieving one solution immediately collapses the other problem. More often, this is not the case.

Consider that for some people, the sound of a baby crying is the sound of a child trying to communicate, and is seen as a sound of joy. To others, the sound of crying is hyperacoustic in nature, and something to be avoided. For the latter, crying is one of the most distressing sounds that can be experienced.

Tinnitus is a noise that is "heard" in the conscious, active part of the brain, and because of this fact, we can always alter at least one of the two problems facing us. *We can almost always change the interpretation of the sound we hear*. It isn't easy, but it is done every day here in therapy. *Changing your interpretation of hearing tinnitus is a key change that **must** be made for your optimal recovery.*

In most cases we can reduce the volume of the tinnitus, and in some cases we can eliminate it completely. "Persistent" improvement in volume reduction is a mid– to long–term task, however. We can begin the process of healing by maintaining

Subdivide your healing goals into two areas.

1. Reduce the volume level.

2. Reduce the level of suffering.

patience and the realization that it will take time to go from the experience of, "this noise is driving me insane" to "this noise is annoying." This is a giant step to accomplish and it is not as easy as saying, "Learn to live with it." Healing will require a realistic expectation that you *will* experience bad days after beginning therapy, and that in the long term, you *will* improve your situation.

It should be obvious by now that a person who experienced SPADE (stress, panic disorder, anxiety, depression, and/or emotional problems) before the onset of tinnitus will find it more difficult to cognitively put a "positive spin" on tinnitus, once onset has occurred. A person who was very happy before the tinnitus onset will find tinnitus reduction an easier process, on average, than a person who was depressed or suffered from panic or anxiety disorders. Therefore, caring for your emotional health is now as important as working with your tinnitus reduction in your healing process. This can be done through self-help, various therapeutic interventions, and psychopharmacology. All of these methods are detailed in the pages just ahead.

> We can almost always change the interpretation of the sound we hear.

Your interpretation of what the tinnitus "means" is very important to your healing. It could be useful to look at your tinnitus as a random event in your life, unrelated to luck, fate, or the will of supernatural beings. It could be useful for you to realize that suffering from tinnitus is a normal and reasonable response to an unwanted stimulus. *If your tinnitus is perceived as random and meaningless, then it is easier for the brain to find other stimuli to pay attention to.* As soon as meaning is attached to a stimulus, it becomes "important" and is recalled (heard) in more contexts. If you believe you have been cursed or are the victim of bad luck, you will want to work through these beliefs and eventually change them to the belief that your noise is simply a random event. The random event will be easier to work through in the therapeutic process. (By the way, scientific reality may determine that tinnitus is not a random event. However, when considering therapeutic improvement, we know from Dr. Martin Seligman's work in optimism and helplessness that approaching challenges like this in the fashion I have described is among the best approach to problems of this nature.)

Once the negative perception of tinnitus has become a "reason" for lifestyle changes such as quitting a job, getting a divorce, or even suicide, psychotherapy, hypnotherapy and pharmacological interventions are strongly indicated. The support of a skilled therapist is very important to people who have considered taking their life. There is no shame in considering suicide because of severe tinnitus. Realize the consideration and take advantage of those who get paid to listen and help you through the tough and trying days of tinnitus suffering.

Caring for your emotional health is now as important as working with your tinnitus reduction in your healing process.

Severe tinnitus is considered the third most difficult malady to live with, following only intractable pain and intractable dizziness. Suicidal thoughts do demand assistance. **It is a sign of emotional strength to ask for help.** The probability for long term tinnitus volume reduction is so great that suicide needs no longer to be a consideration. A multi-modal approach to your healing may not eliminate the noise completely, but in time, the probability is high for reducing the volume to a level that is tolerable.

There is an interesting benefit to experiencing tinnitus that is "born in depression." As the depression is addressed (or any element of SPADE) and improved or "lifted," the tinnitus tends to follow the depression. In other words, once an individual escapes from depression, tinnitus becomes less perceptible. In some cases, remission is around the corner.

Tinnitus and Your Emotional Brain

Tinnitus, "the noise," is running through your brain on hundreds of highways called neural pathways. These neural pathways may be visualized as roads between brain cells. The "intersections" in the brain's highways are called synapses. These intersections do not actually touch each other. The open space between the cell arms is called the synapse. The highways are made up of axons and dendrites. (It's not necessary that you know this, but it's interesting.). Information is sent from one cell to another via a neurotransmitter, much like a cellular phone call; and the "phones" are not connected by wires. We'll talk a little more about these neurons and neurotransmitters in a moment.

First, it will be useful for you to understand some ways people get depressed, feel stressed, become panicked, or experience anxiety, and, how all of this relates to tinnitus.

In 1995, I coined an acronym, S.P.A.D.E (or SPADE)., to represent the following:

    S – Stress
    P – Panic Disorder
    A – Anxiety

D – Depression

E – Emotional Challenges

Research into tinnitus suffering shows that the "ingredients" of SPADE tend to predispose people to tinnitus (and other somatics as well). SPADE is a significant set of variables in determining who will experience suffering from tinnitus and who will not. SPADE is most likely a significant variable in who experiences tinnitus after exposure to loud noise or other physical stimuli. *The emotional part of our brain, it appears, is critical in the experience, suffering, and relief from tinnitus.*

There may be a stigma that goes with this line of thinking. If we acknowledge an emotional component to the onset, and later to suffering of tinnitus, we acknowledge that it is at least tangentially something that could be "mistaken" as a "mental illness." However, since such terms are useless in the healing process, we will not concern ourselves with such labels. You can call anxiety a "brain cold" and "depression" a case of the "mind flu." The name doesn't matter; getting better does. Our objective will always be the reduction and/or elimination of tinnitus. Period.

Tinnitus suffering is positively correlated to all the elements of SPADE. The emotional part of our brain, it appears, is critical in the experience, suffering, and relief from tinnitus. For now, consider the insidious relationship between brain chemistry and stress, stress and depression, and all of these emotional states and tinnitus. In SPADE, "the first factor" seems to be stress.

In 1993, Dr. G. W. Brown wrote that he discovered **84 percent of a large sample of depressed patients had experienced severe stress in the preceding year,** compared to 32 percent of control subjects. Drs. Anisman and Zacharko have suggested that the depletion of certain neurotransmitters (e.g., of dopamine, serotonin, and norepinephrine) that are associated with stress may leave an individual sensitized to subsequent stress and thus less capable of coping with it. They *view the inability to cope effectively with stress as a major predisposing factor in depression* (*Biopsychology*, 1997, Allyn and Bacon Press).

Important studies involving patients with tinnitus reveal that depression precedes a significantly large numbers of tinnitus cases. People not suffering from depression develop tinnitus less regularly.

Therefore, for at least a significantly large percentage of the patients suffering from tinnitus, we know that many were predisposed to tinnitus by depression and, before that, severe stress. Further, we know from various drug studies that anti-anxiety medications *(Xanax)* and anti-depressants (**Pamelor**) have been shown to reduce tinnitus volume in a significant number of patients. (76 percent and 43 percent respectively, compared to 4 percent for a placebo.)

Anti-convulsants like **Klonopin** have also been shown to be successful in reducing tinnitus in large numbers of patients. Klonopin is regularly prescribed for individuals who suffer from epilepsy and/or related seizures. Later in this book we will discuss research that has been done into just how much of what drug to use and when to take medications with a medical doctor's prescription.)

The beneficial effects for tinnitus reduction and distress reduction by these medications offer us our first clues as to the causes and potential elimination of tinnitus.

For many people with tinnitus, negative emotional experiences play a pivotal role in onset, suffering, and later, relief from tinnitus. Severe tinnitus challenges the emotional stability of even the most resilient individual. Tinnitus is far more than a simple hearing disorder. Tinnitus is a complex intermingling of deficient brain chemistry, phantom auditory perception, cell receptor damage, and/or negative emotional experiences (among other variables). Tinnitus sounds may be similar from person to person, but the cause, onset, volume, and experience of that tinnitus can be very different. One modality of reducing tinnitus may work for some but *it is becoming clear that a multi-modal approach to tinnitus reduction is indicated for most individuals.*

Stress, depression, panic disorder, and anxiety are like fertilized soil for a farmer. The farmer planting the crops can be likened to the physical stimulus that causes the tinnitus and makes it persist (grow), while in most people, without the fertile soil, it only lasts a period of time. Once the tinnitus is "planted" in the brain of stressed or depressed individuals, it grows and soon plateaus in volume.

The brain initially becomes aware of this noise and initially does not like the noise. The part of the brain that probably detects the potential negative impact of this noise is the amygdala. It does this by comparing the sound of the noise to other noises the brain has experienced in the past, then determining whether action should be taken or not against the sound. (Unfortunately the amygdala cannot help us take action in reducing the noise.)

As the brain becomes accustomed to having the noise around, the noise is accepted as part of the daily experience of life. Tinnitus is often perceived as a threat to survival and the amygdala demands that it be found when the conscious mind notices it is "not there." (Have you noticed that when you awaken from a nap your tinnitus volume increases? For many, this is your brain's way of trying to keep you alive. The tinnitus is as persistent as breathing and, as with breathing, the brain will make sure the noise is detected if the tinnitus is correlated to a survival issue in some way.)

The brain does not think that tinnitus is "good." It simply is a survival issue. An intruding sound has been detected and a "sound loop" is created in the neural pathways that keeps the tinnitus perception intact. Long after the physical stimulation for the tinnitus is gone (a loud concert for example), the tinnitus persists. The brain continues to find the noise. This is what is meant when it is said that tinnitus is psychosomatic in nature, even though the tinnitus onset was physical. *Psychosomatic means that there is a significant emotional cause to a physical medical problem.* In tinnitus, this is often, but not always the case. You will soon discover that this relationship works to your advantage when you begin your daily regimen to reduce tinnitus volume and distress. This is good news for the sufferer.

The continuation of noise (persistent tinnitus) is often not "necessary." If there is no evidence of significant sensorineural hearing loss, then the probability of tinnitus remission is significantly increased. The brain can be re-wired and re-programmed to stop playing the endless looping of tinnitus tapes. (Those with sensorineural hearing loss can also experience remission of tinnitus, but in our clinical experience, it is less often.)

Tinnitus can be experienced in one of three general locations.

1. Central (In the head)
2. Aurium (Unilateral- One Side)

3. Binaural (Bilateral- Both Sides)

Surprisingly, the subjective experience does not necessarily reflect the location of the generation of the tinnitus. The best way to determine the location of the generation of the tinnitus is with a furosemide infusion.

Research reported in 1996 by Drs. Shulman, Aronson, and Strashun seems to reveal *three distinct forms of central tinnitus*. Central tinnitus, as opposed to unilateral or bilateral tinnitus, is important to understand in reducing tinnitus volume because by central we are really "saying brain." SPECT Imaging of brain and tinnitus was accomplished with some of the following apparent neurotologic and neurologic implications. (Note: This is my interpretation of very technical research based on Shulman, Aronson, Strashun, et. al.)

Tinnitus that is of central origin (not in the ears) seems to be of three general categories.

(A) **Cerebrovascular disease** where there is reduced blood flow to the cerebral hemisphere. (This may result in a stroke by the individual.)

(B) **Neurogenerative disorders** and associated dementia. Alzheimer's is an example; palsy would be another.

(C) **Neuropsychiatric disorders** such as dementia, schizophrenia, and affective disorder of depression. It is speculated that there may be a link between thought disorders present in schizophrenia and pathological sites in the left temporal lobe. A key for our discussion is the fact that SPECT studies of affective disorder show an overall decrease in regional rCBF especially in the frontal lobes. In depression the CBF seems to be normalized with clinical patient improvement.

*It appears that there may be a creation of a
paradoxical auditory memory center, by the tinnitus,
in the hippocampal amygdala complex, and other
portions of the limbic system may result in varying
degrees of abnormality in affect ranging from mild
anxiety to severe depression.*

The significance of re-wiring the brain, as in the case of Derrick, appears as important as pharmacological intervention when considering this data.

Noise and Negative Emotions:
Paired For A Time

"Negative emotions" such as fear, depression, and anxiety are paired with the sound of tinnitus for most tinnitus sufferers. Whether the individual experienced these emotions prior to the "onset" of tinnitus, is not critical to volume reduction. What is vital is understanding how tinnitus and negative emotions are paired in the brain, so we can unhook them once and for all.

If we hope to "re-wire" the brain, we must know where and how to do the wiring. Therefore, we need to consider exactly what happens when we "hear" tinnitus. Once we understand how tinnitus is heard, then we can begin our job discovering what will help most people gain significant relief from the incessant noises.

For people who do not like listening to the noise we call tinnitus, the brain experiences ongoing stimulus/response patterns, over and over and over again. Day after day and month after month the cyclical experience occurs. The good news is that this pattern and cycle are correctable for most.

We know more about how negative emotions such as fear and noise are paired in the brain than about any other sensory stimulus and response. For years, scientists have paired noises with electrical shocks to create fear in laboratory animals. Scientists have dissected the brains of these animals, and we know the highways (neural pathways) that fear travels through the brain. We know where these distressing noises are heard and experienced. In other words, we know enough now, at the beginning of the 21st century, to *create* tinnitus and fear in animals. We also know, subjectively, what it is like to experience both tinnitus and the fear–related emotions of depression, stress, anxiety, and panic disorder.

The tinnitus sufferer is someone whose brain detects the noise and then interprets the noise as dangerous or threatening, in some manner. This evolutionary response saves the lives of those who have a brain tumor. A simple MRI scan can find the smallest neuroma, and surgery can save the life of someone who simply heard tinnitus caused by pressure on the eighth nerve. This is, of course, the exception rather than the rule in the tinnitus experience, however.

Humans are probably born with two fears, and only two. The fear of falling is one, and the fear of loud noises is the other. Severe tinnitus falls into the category of the second. This innate fear of loud sounds is very difficult, but not impossible to unhook. Until we begin to unhook fear from the distressing noise, no relief is likely to be experienced.

In addition to the two inborn human phobias, we know that disorders such as anxiety, phobias, and obsessive compulsive disorders also tend to be predisposed genetically. This combination makes for a powerful recipe when tinnitus onsets. Overcoming genetic tendencies in experience or behavior is always challenging. Yet challenges are meant to be overcome. The challenge of tinnitus reduction is a great one, and it is accomplished every day by people around the world. Understanding the connection between emotions and suffering from tinnitus is critical to our solving this most challenging puzzle.

You will probably find this hard to believe, but it is true: *About two–thirds of all individuals who experience moderate tinnitus experience no suffering from the noise(s).* These people seek no medical or mental health attention, and have no significant negative emotional responses to the noises they hear. This is going to be another goal you will want to achieve.

Volume and Frequency: How Do They Relate to Suffering?

The best studies on the correlation between volume, frequency, distress, and suffering were done in Australia by Jane Henry, Ph.D. and Peter Wilson, Ph.D., and reported in the *International Journal of Tinnitus* in 1995. My interpretation of their research (and other similar studies) is summarized below.

■ Anxiety is probably the only significant emotional effect of tinnitus for those who "cope" well with tinnitus.

■ Depression is a common emotional effect of tinnitus for those who "cope" poorly with tinnitus and suffer from it. (The neurobiological differences between those who suffer and those who do not will be discussed in the next section.)

■ Extremely loud tinnitus is correlated to distress.

■ Moderate levels of tinnitus are not correlated to distress.

■ More severely distressed patients experienced elevated levels of depression.

- High–distress subjects report engaging in more dysfunctional thinking about their tinnitus.
- Dysfunctional thinking tends to be specific to tinnitus, and not generalized to life issues.
- High–distress patients tend to experience more general dysfunctional thinking when compared to lower–distress patients.
- Tinnitus is not necessarily a depressive disorder.
- Some people are severely debilitated by tinnitus.

So what is it that causes one person with tinnitus of 45 dB at 6,000 hz to be severely debilitated by the noise, and another person with identical volume and frequency to find the noise largely irrelevant? The answer is in the brain, the emotional brain.

Tinnitus Suffering and the Emotional Brain

Joseph LeDoux, professor of neuroscience at New York University proposes that "anxiety disorders come about when the fear system breaks loose from the cortical controls that usually keep the primitive impulses—the wild things in us, at bay…."

"Anxiety," he says, "is the result of traumatic learning experiences. Since traumatic learning involves, at least in part, fear conditioning, it is possible that similar brain mechanisms contribute to pathogenic anxiety in humans…"

This proposition is useful in understanding the powerful link between tinnitus and emotions.

The tinnitus sufferer's brain first experiences tinnitus either in the ear, normally from the cochlea, or in the temporal lobe of the brain. In either case, the sound that is produced triggers a pathway of fear or a similar emotion (depression, disgust, frustration, annoyance, anxiety, panic). This emotion races to the **brainstem**. The brainstem is the part of the brain on which the cerebral hemispheres rest; in general, it regulates reflex activities that are critical for survival, including heart rate and respiration among others.

Having reached the brainstem, the emotion immediately moves out to the **thalamus**. (Our interest is specifically in the auditory thalamus, which acts as a relay station, sending acoustic signals from the receptors in the ears to the auditory cortex. Laboratory animals that have had the auditory thalamus lesioned, are unable to experience fear with sounds.

From the thalamus, a couple of significant paths split off. A small bundle of projections leads to the **amygdala** and its neighbor in the brain, the **hippocampus**. (There are two of each of these brain components. The hippocampus is involved with registering and making sense of patterns of perception. It puts memories into context, which is important to emotional meaning and interpretation. The hippocampus allows you to distinguish between a lion in your backyard and a lion safely tucked away behind bars in a zoo. The hippocampus leads to sophisticated computational power.)

A much larger bundle of projections goes to the **auditory cortex** in the **temporal lobe**, where sounds are sorted, evaluated, considered, and saved.

The hippocampus quickly decides how important the tinnitus is, and the auditory cortex does a more extensive evaluation. Is it louder than normal? Is it more annoying? Is this tinnitus something to worry more about than yesterday's? Is it getting worse?

If the brain is emotionally stimulated (fear, anxiety, panic, depression, stress) by the noise, the amygdala pulls a "fire alarm" in the brain that activates the **hypothalamus** (located just below the thalamus), The hypothalamus plays an important role in the regulation of several motivated behaviors. It exerts its effects, in part, by regulating the release of hormones from the pituitary gland, the brainstem, and the **autonomic nervous system,** the division of the peripheral nervous system that regulates the body's inner environment. The autonomic nervous system is composed of afferent nerves that carry sensory signals from internal organs to the central nervous system, and efferent nerves that carry motor signals from the CNS to internal organs. (Afferent means going toward, efferent means coming from.)

The hypothalamus releases a hormone called corticopin–releasing hormone (CRH), which gives us the flight or fight experience by releasing numerous other hormones into the brain and the body. The survival response is very useful when there is an immediate threat to our well being. When there is no such threat, the release of this important hormone can be devastating to our long–term physical, emotional, and mental health.

A great deal of "negative" intra-brain communication is going on at this point. One pathway from the amygdala leads to the locus cereuleus in the brainstem noted above. This part of the brain manufactures and disperses **norepinephrine** (a monoamine neurotransmitter) into the brain. Norepinephrine essentially heightens the sensitivity of the overall reactivity of the brain areas that receive it, making the sensory circuits more sensitive. "Norepinephrine suffuses the cortex, the brainstem, and the limbic system itself, in essence setting the brain on edge." (Daniel Goleman, Emotional Intelligence, 1996)

A person begins to experience many of the normal stress responses now. Shortened breaths, slower respiration, higher blood pressure, and faster heart rate are all possible.

Meanwhile, back in the brain, the amygdala, "along with the interconnected hippocampus, directs the cells that send key neurotransmitters, for example, to trigger releases of **dopamine** (another small molecule monoamine neurotransmitter), that leads to the riveting of attention on the source of your fear—the strange sounds—and put your muscles at readiness to react accordingly." (Goleman, 1996)

Experiencing this set of actions and reactions is enough to put a person in a physical state equivalent to fighting a battle on the battlefield. This battle, unfortunately, is fought within the mind, brain, and body of the tinnitus sufferer. The continual release of the powerful hormones suppresses the immune system, and over time the sufferer's health begins to decline in numerous areas. The emotional stability of the sufferer is on edge, and it is sometimes a miracle that a person with severe tinnitus makes it through the day.

The emotional response to tinnitus, when constantly paired with tinnitus noise, makes the bond closer as each day passes. This occurs because the loop between the subcortical amygdala and the thalamus is faster and shorter than the road from the auditory thalamus to the auditory cortex, back to the amygdala, sharing better evaluated information.

The constant influx of stress hormones through the brain and body is enough to create emotional problems such as generalized anxiety, panic disorder, and depression. It appears that the hippocampus (discussed above) can literally shrink when under too much stress. It is critical to reverse this situation as early as possible. Meanwhile, stress enhances the ability of the amygdala to function. It thrives on such experiences. Unfortunately, it is just such activity that assists in the creation of pairing negative emotions and a stimulus such as tinnitus.

In other words, it is critical to address both the cortical and subcortical responses to tinnitus in order to quiet the noise and reduce the emotional response. One significant therapeutic event that must occur for the tinnitus sufferer is the complete cognitive understanding that subjective idiopathic tinnitus (for lack of a better term) is completely acceptable and unworthy of attention. The conscious mind (hippocampal system) is best dealt with in psychotherapy. The unconscious mind (amygdala system) is best dealt with in hypnotherapy and by utilizing various medications. Hypnotherapy and pharmacological interventions work best for one part of the re-wiring process. Tinnitus Habituation Therapy is another vital element which will be discussed later.

"The amygdala is like the hub of a wheel. It receives low-level inputs from sensory-specific regions of the thalamus, higher level information from sensory-specific cortex, and still higher level (sensory independent) information about the general situation from the hippocampal formation. The amygdala is able to process the emotional significance of individual stimuli as well as complex situations. The amygdala is, in essence, involved in the appraisal of emotional meaning. It is where trigger stimuli do their triggering.

"...It is easy to imagine how malfunctions of the amygdala and its neural partners might lead to emotional disorders...." (Joseph LeDoux, The Emotional Brain, 1996).

The amygdala is the heart of the unconscious mind. This may explain why hypnotherapy is effective in unhooking tinnitus from emotion. It is certainly true that the number of receptor sites in this region of the brain that are benzodiazepine friendly makes a good case for the use of anti-anxiety medications in the uncoupling of tinnitus and emotion, and indeed extinguishing the fear–related responses (depression, anxiety, panic, post traumatic stress disorder, etc.) from the tinnitus stimulus.

One process utilized in hypnotherapy is presenting the tinnitus sufferer with various negative stimuli that the sufferer is likely to have experienced in early childhood before the hippocampus was fully developed. Responses are exhibited with ideomotor (finger) signals. The amygdala normally does not have specific memories of specific events. It does, however, have specific responses to general stimuli in order to "protect" the individual by detecting danger.

As you have learned, for some people, tinnitus is an irrelevant noise. For other people, tinnitus is detected by the amygdala as a threatening and imminent danger. Most people with tinnitus fall somewhere in between these two extremes. *Through hypnotherapy, we can re-educate the amygdala. After discovering responses that may have caused the brain to generalize fear responses to tinnitus, we can recondition the stimuli to become irrelevant and fear resistant. This new response hooks tinnitus to another response that may be verbalized as "a little annoying."* It can be physiologically measured using galvanic skin response, but it is difficult to describe in linguistic terms. It is not a simple process, nor quick; but it is effective.

There are more steps in reducing tinnitus volume beyond simply utilizing hypnotherapy or benzodiazepines (a class of GABA agonists with anxiolytic, sedative, and anticonvulsant properties) to effectively extinguish the conditioned emotional responses to tinnitus. The process will also require significant lifestyle changes. The brain can return to its bad habits if we don't alter our lifestyles by reducing the stressful elements in our life, creating solutions to depression, and making major changes in that environment that impacts our emotions.

Lifestyle changes are normally difficult to implement, and in the short term, the good news is that the medication Xanax (alprazolam) will help raise thresholds for anxiety, fear, depression and negative emotion. As discussed previously, medications like Xanax work, in part, by binding to the benzodiazepine receptors throughout the brain. These receptors facilitate the effect of the inhibitory neurotransmitter, **GABA** (one of four amino acids that are considered to be neurotransmitters by most experts in the field). Increasing inhibition means increasing the threshold for anxiety. For people who suffer from tinnitus, this can be a large piece of the healing puzzle. The action of Xanax (and other benzodiazepines) in the amygdala appears particularly significant, since it reduces the excitatory transmission. Pairing pharmacological intervention with hypnotherapy and psychotherapy, the probability of extinguishing negative emotional responses to tinnitus is dramatically increased. As the sound(s) becomes unimportant, the brain begins to ignore them. Sometimes this can result in tinnitus remitting.

The same, or a similar, mechanism that allows for the anxiety threshold to heighten by increasing inhibition of GABA also appears to be highly relevant to maintaining tinnitus and the emotional response to tinnitus.

"It is hypothesized that a fundamental function of the amygdala–hippocampal structures is the establishment of a paradoxical auditory memory for tinnitus. It is a result of alteration in auditory masking found in all tinnitus patients. A paradoxical memory for an aberrant auditory signal, i.e., tinnitus, is considered to be the initial process in the transition of sensory to the affect component. Underlying mechanisms are hypothesized to exist and to be highlighted by a diminution of inhibition mediated by gamma aminobutryic acid (GABA), due to disconnection from excitatory (glutamate) inputs. Blockage of GABA mediated inhibition results in Tinnitogenesis, an epileptiform auditory phenomena." *(Final Common Pathway for Tinnitus – The Medial Temporal Lobe System,* Abraham Shulman, M.D., 1995.)

There is no other logical explanation for a final common pathway for tinnitus that coincidentally produces an aberrant auditory phenomenon and the powerful emotional responses experienced in relationship to tinnitus. We cannot underestimate the significance of Shulman's work in understanding tinnitus and how it relates to treatment and therapy.

I have worked in depth and in great detail with over 1000 clients with tinnitus in the past three years. Shulman and his associates worked with 4,000 patients in the previous twenty years. His work merits careful consideration before we move on to non-central tinnitus.

Shulman speculates that there may be a lesion in the brain of individuals with central tinnitus (tinnitus that emanates from the brain and not necessarily the ear). My personal experience with such tinnitus, and that of my clients, leads me to believe that if there is such a lesion, the effects of the lesion can be regularly bypassed and do not demand hearing tinnitus all of the time.

Shulman also has discovered in over 90 percent of all individuals he has examined using advanced SPECT imaging of the brain, side to side perfusion asymmetries involving **the medial temporal lobe system** (MTLS); frontal, temporal, and parietal areas of the brain.

Neuroscientists believe that the MTLS, which includes the amygdala, hippocampus, and other portions of the brain, is the location where memory and stress meet. The MTLS, which is part of the limbic lobe, encircles the upper brain stem.

Returning to Le Doux's research for a moment, we can consider the fact that Le Doux has identified a neuroanatomical subcortical processing circuit (i.e., thalmo-amygdala), in which **the emotional significance of an auditory stimulus can be learned, stored in memory, and be expressed in body physiology by the autonomic nervous system**. (Le Doux, *Journal of Neuroscience*, 1990).

Shulman has hypothesized that sensory systems and emotions are linked by memory (Shulman, Strashun, Goldstein, Afryie; 4th International Tinnitus Seminar Transactions, 1991).

For the lay reader, *the key to understanding tinnitus is realizing that you are hearing an ever-present memory.* This "memory" is similar, if not identical, to a Pavlovian conditioned response that loops endlessly: Hear Tinnitus ⇨ Feel Depressed ⇨ Hear Tinnitus ⇨ Feel Depressed and on and on. Another loop that may have been conditioned is Hear Tinnitus ⇨ Feel Anxious ⇨ Hear Tinnitus ⇨ Feel Anxious. Eventually there is a question of "Which came first: the chicken or the egg?". The link between emotion and tinnitus is so powerful and so bonded in the brain that the loop is tight and spins endlessly. Shulman calls this kind of feedback loop, "masking," not to be confused with the therapy for tinnitus called tinnitus masking. Shulman considers tinnitus to be "an auditory error, i.e., a defect in the ability of the masking neurons to function normally." (Shulman, 1995)

Dr. Shulman publishes updates on tinnitus research twice annually in his publication, *The International Tinnitus Journal*. The *ITJ* is the best publication in the world for keeping current on tinnitus research.

A key objective of this book is to help you, the reader, replicate the experience of millions of people who experience tinnitus but do not suffer from it. Those people who hear tinnitus but do not suffer have had no internal emotional (amygdala) negative evaluations of the sound(s) itself. This is one goal I would like you to consider setting for yourself.

People who find tinnitus to be irrelevant rarely notice the noise, since it is not picked up as important by the subcortical (emotional) brain.

In my experience with hundreds of clients, these feedback loops can be unhooked, or at least loosened, in most cases. As you can imagine, the process will take time, and the path will be fraught with difficulties that test your will and determination. You will learn a few self–help techniques later in this book, but you will eventually contact a skilled hypnotherapist and a medical doctor to assist you with proper medications to nurture the process.

For many people, the sound of tinnitus is not generated, at least initially, in the brain, but in the inner ear. For these people the mechanism of generation is often the emissions of damaged hair cells in the cochlea. These sounds are interminably being generated through the auditory nerve into the brainstem for the same looping that was discussed previously. In these cases, we must also work on volume reduction in the inner ear. In addition, even if we unhook the stimulus tinnitus from the negative emotional responses, we realize that they can easily pair up again at a later date. Another very big challenge is about to be faced head on.

Tinnitus and Your Inner Ear

In this section, we will not discuss in great detail types of tinnitus that are related to typical otological events and disorders (ear problems). Here we want to consider what is normally missed with standard audiological instruments. A competent Ear, Nose, and Throat doctor (ENT) will detect and treat any presenting ear problems for you. This portion of the chapter, for the most part, will show you what the ENT's instruments do not pick up. Then, if initial treatment fails, you can share this information with your ENT, otologist or other medical professional.

Tinnitus can be considered an auditory perception, for our discussion in this section. Once a "physical" cause for the tinnitus has been eliminated, it is useful to view tinnitus in this fashion. We can then treat the noise as an auditory perception. It is neither good nor bad. It simply is something that is perceived. If you are fortunate enough to have tinnitus that is phantom auditory perception, you have several options for treatment.

Possible Causes of Tinnitus

Ototoxic drugs are drugs that can create problems in hearing and can also cause tinnitus. Ototoxic means "ear poison." Many people who have come to see me had used drugs that were ototoxic in nature up until the onset of their tinnitus. Ibuprofin is an over–the–counter medication that is anti-inflammatory in nature. Anti-inflammatory drugs are among the most common offenders that I have noted on my intake charts as tinnitus creators. Naproxen is another common offending drug. Another set of common offenders are antibiotics. Not all antibiotics are ototoxic in nature, but many are. (If the name of your antibiotic ends in "mycin," look out! You have a suspect.) The good news about anti-inflammatory drugs is that when you stop taking the medications, there is an excellent chance the tinnitus will quiet shortly thereafter. The bad news is that in the case of antibiotics, the damage to the hearing and tinnitus is more than likely going to be permanent. (This was my four–year old daughter's experience, and the cause of sensorineural hearing loss.)

Less common, in my experience, but regularly noted in studies and research papers, are diuretics, oral contraceptives, quinine, street drugs, alcohol, over–the–counter drugs, nicotine, anti-inflammatory drugs, some anti-anxiety drugs, and some anti-depressants, such as Elavil.

If you are taking these kinds of drugs and have tinnitus that is bothering you, it would make sense to ask your doctor for other alternatives, if possible. *Even aspirin can induce tinnitus!*

The good news for aspirin–induced tinnitus is that it usually recedes when the intake of aspirin is stopped.

Other kinds of drugs that have been known to cause tinnitus are salicylates. **Salicylates** are used in the production of aspirin and many other pharmaceuticals. Interestingly enough, salicylates are also used in the preservation of certain kinds of foods! The challenge, of course, is finding a specific offending agent may be causing the tinnitus. Pay close attention to your aspirin intake. An aspirin each day for the heart is probably a good thing. Ten aspirins per day can cause tinnitus, and, in some cases, hearing loss. Significant decreases of salt and sugar from the diet may be useful in reducing tinnitus. It is important to watch your intake of cholesterol and triglycerides, along with anything that may result in poor blood circulation. Check with your physician before making any changes in your diet or medications.

Diabetes and hyperinsulinemia are often linked to the onset of tinnitus. The reason, most likely, is reduced blood flow to the ear area. The hair cells do not get their full supply of "nutrients." Most diabetics are already aware of the role of diet and health, and I would echo your medical practitioner's advice to you. One recent study indicated that 84 percent of all people with subjective idiopathic tinnitus had hyperinsulinemia. ("Hyperinsulinemia: The Common Denominator of Subjective Idiopathic Tinnitus and Other Idiopathic Central and Peripheral Neurootological Disorders;" Joseph Kraft, M.D., *International Tinnitus Journal,* 1995.)

Eating several small carbohydrate based meals throughout the day may help those suffering from tinnitus due to diabetes and hyperinsulinemia.

Physical trauma was previously noted as a common trigger of tinnitus. The entire inner ear area is very delicate, and it takes very little for you to "get your bell rung." Unfortunately, sometimes the bells keep ringing. The next chapter will include methods of reducing tinnitus, including tinnitus that is traumatically induced.

Ear wax can cause both tinnitus and the inability to hear. Have your doctor check your ears and *carefully* remove ear wax from your ear if it appears necessary.

Barotrauma is damage to the ear caused by sudden abnormal pressure relationships affecting the external, middle, and/or inner ear. It is infrequent as a cause of tinnitus, but when it does occur, it may be associated with pain, hearing loss, perforated ear drum, bleeding from the ear, and/or dizziness (suggesting possible leakage of fluid from the middle ear). Barotrauma can occur in connection with water sports (including diving) as well as during rapid altitude changes, such as those sometimes occurring during flight in under-pressurized planes.

One client I worked with in 1997 had no tinnitus and only some hearing loss before an airplane flight. After the flight, she was profoundly deaf, and her tinnitus volume was estimated at over 90 dB.

Other physiological causes of tinnitus include **Meniere's Disease, allergies, high or low blood pressure**, and otosclerosis, among others. **Otosclerosis** is a condition of the ear that is often correctable by a surgery called a *stapedectomy*. This surgery removes the stapes (the innermost of the three small bones of the ear, also called the stirrup bone), which the surgeon then replaces with a small wire or other similar prosthesis. This operation has been in existence for some 35 years and is normally successful in restoring hearing, but it does not have excellent success in reducing the volume of tinnitus. Otosclerosis patients would probably do well to utilize sodium fluoride to help reduce or eliminate tinnitus. The recommended dosage is 40mg/day taken with Vitamin D.

Having considered causes of tinnitus that are readily diagnosable by your medical professional, let us now turn to tinnitus that is probably generated in the ear. The major type of tinnitus discussed below is cochlear synaptic tinnitus. This common type of tinnitus is much more difficult to specifically diagnose, and below I discuss the medications and vitamins being used to treat it which, hopefully, will help you understand more about the this type of tinnitus.

Research reported from 1995–1997 reveals that **caroverine,** a glutamate antagonist, is successful at reducing tinnitus volume Glutamate is an amino acid and the brain's most prevalent excitatory neurotransmitter. Glutamate is very important to smooth brain functioning, but too much or too little glutamate can cause a variety of problems.

In the ear, signals between the inner hair cells and the cochlear afferent are transmitted by means of the mediator glutamate. Glutamate excites three different receptor subtypes in the postsynaptic membrane of the afferent cochlear neuron. According to tinnitus researchers in Austria and Switzerland (Ehrenberger, Denk, and Felix):

A disturbed interplay of these receptor subgroups
causes pathological excitation states which are
perceived subjectively as cochlear synaptic tinnitus,
associated with latent or manifest inner ear disorders
(which are themselves caused by glutamate

intoxication) is the basis for receptor pharmacological concepts for the treatment of this very common form of tinnitus: selective glutamate antagonists should be capable of restoring the physiological relationship between the different activities of the three receptor subgroups. The growing number of clinical successes in tinnitus therapy confirm the working hypotheses upon which these therapeutic concepts are based.

The three researchers have more to offer about forms of tinnitus generated from the inner ear.

*Tinnitus as an isolated phenomenon appears to have a particular cause, namely the disturbed interplay of glutamate receptor subtypes which are independent of one another and which have been damaged to different degrees. This disturbed interplay modulates the spontaneous activity of the nerve in such a way that pathological **depolarizations** (process of decreasing the membrane's potential) occur, which stimulate the excitation effects of sounds and are misinterpreted centrally as signals from peripheral sounds.*

The researchers tell us the goal with the individual with this form of tinnitus is to "protect the receptors from excessive excitation and in the case of tinnitus, to restore equilibrium of excitations between the different receptor subtypes."

Caroverine, which has yet to be approved in the United States, appears to be a useful medication for treating cochlear–synaptic tinnitus. Caroverine seems to antagonize the membrane response to glutamate, acting as a guardian and stabilizer. The drug Tinnex (caroverine hydrochloride), available in countries like Japan, Austria, Spain, and Denmark among others, is the brand name of the generic. Phafag, the drug's manufacturer, states that the drug is indicated in acute and chronic tinnitus (metabolic inner ear tinnitus), explicable in terms of the cochlear synaptic tinnitus model, e.g. loss of hearing in old age (presbycusis) , sudden loss of hearing, unilateral or bilateral sensorineural auditory dysfunction. In such cases, 66 percent of trial subjects experienced a 25 percent or more reduction in their tinnitus volume. Tinnitus in middle ear diseases, mechanical cochlear tinnitus (e.g. blast injury), retrocochlear tinnitus are not of cochlear–synaptic etiology and have to be ruled out.

Phafag adds that,

> *Our concept is based on the working hypothesis that glutamate, known to be among the most important neurotransmitters in the central nervous system, is the most likely transmitter substance in the afferent cochlear synapse. On the subsynaptic membrane, two different types of receptors, which work as a dual receptor system (NMDA, non-NMDA) are stimulated by glutamate.*
>
> *The dual receptor system is responsible for a typical pattern of depolarization. Under pathological conditions, spontaneous receptor-dependent depolarization patterns mimic sound–induced patterns, which differ from the normally irregular pattern and are perceived by the patient as tinnitus. This may occur under excessive stimulation of the*

receptors, for example, when the transmitter
glutamate develops neurotoxine activity.

Assuming the minimal side effects noted in the literature, it is this author's hope that Tinnex and Spasmium (see below) will soon be requested by enough tinnitus sufferers in the United States that the drug is eventually released here.

Recent research indicates that blocking NMDA receptors in the amygdala prevents fear conditioning. (Fanselow and Kim, 1994) The good news is that the use of medications blocking NMDA receptors in the amygdala may reduce tinnitus distress. There is a caveat. Conditioning is another word for learning, and learning involves memory. Therefore, even though physical side effects are likely to be insignificant, using medications that block NMDA receptors should be done with very careful supervision by a medical professional.

Simultaneous research to the caroverine studies in Europe seem to show a potential benefit for many sufferers using low doses of *magnesium* to assist in reducing tinnitus. There is some additional research that may also give hope for *zinc* in reducing tinnitus volume, for reasons similar to magnesium. There is speculation that the drug **memantine** may also reduce tinnitus because of its glutamate antagonism.

On another speculative note, calcium channel blockers may also assist some tinnitus sufferers in volume reduction because of the related chemical actions noted above. When glutamate binds to the NMDA receptors of a cell that has just been fired, an action potential, the magnesium block of the NMDA receptor is removed and calcium flows in. The relationships are speculative and may be worthy of consideration by others with greater knowledge of the brain's chemistry than this author.

The drug **Spasmium (generic: caroverine) has been shown to be effective in reducing 66 percent of patients with cochlear synaptic tinnitus**. It appears that diagnoses are not certain, even with thorough screenings. It is thought this drug will work best for people who experience loss of hearing in old age, sudden loss of hearing, unilateral or bilateral sensorineural auditory dysfunction. Dosages vary from individual to individual because of the sensitivity of cell receptors. The usage of caroverine should eventually provide a critical complement to anti-anxiety, anti-depressants, and anti-convulsants in treating tinnitus pharmacologically. The importance of research reported in Austria and Switzerland cannot be understated. Spasmium is available in Austria, Switzerland, and Japan and possibly other countries. The curious reader can refer to the following: *Neuropharmacology,* Vol. 31, No. 12, 1992. Acta Otolaryngol (Stockh) 1995, 115: 236–240. *Otorhinolarynoglogia Nova* 1995, 148-152.

Tinnitus and Your TMJ

If you place your finger in each ear then open your mouth wide, you will feel your temperomandibular joint. As you feel this joint, you sense that it is directly linked to the ear, and indeed it is. (The ear drum is linked to the TMJ by the sphenomandibular ligament.) When the TMJ becomes arthritic, worn, or dysfunctional in any way, the individual can be said to have TMJ Disorder (TMJD or TMD). Symptoms of TMJD are numerous in many individuals. They can include grinding of teeth, misalignment of the jaw and/or teeth, and clicking sounds when opening and closing the mouth. Other common symptoms include headaches, neck pain, and sometimes dizziness. There are many symptoms.

One test that you can do at home is to clench your teeth. If it changes the sound or volume of your tinnitus then there is likely to be a relationship between TMJD and the tinnitus. If this is the case, then self hypnosis audio tapes dealing with relaxation and stress reduction will be especially useful for you.

An epidemiological study reported in Sweden confirms the relationship of tinnitus and TMD "The presence of tinnitus was significantly and positively correlated with reports of neck pain and TMJ–clicking...The presence of hyperacusis was significantly and positively correlated with reports of bruxism, headache, jaw stiffness/tiredness, neck pain, tinnitus, and TMJ–clicking." ("Hyperacusis, Tinnitus, Headache, Temporomandibular Disorders and Amalgam Fillings – An Epidemiological Study," Barbara Rubinstein, Margareta Ahlqwist, and Calle Bengtsoon. Fifth International Tinnitus Seminar, 1995)

Between the brain and ear dysfunctions we have already noted, it would seem that we would have discussed all the key elements in diagnosing and treating tinnitus. As noted earlier in this book, the relationship between tinnitus and a person's Temporomandibular joint (TMJ) is significant in altering the volume or frequency of tinnitus in about a third of all tinnitus sufferers I have worked with. Approximately one–third of people who suffer from tinnitus experience TMJ–Disorder in a manner that is significant to hearing and/or suffering from tinnitus. This third of the tinnitus suffering population can normally manipulate the sound, pitch, and/or volume of their tinnitus by manipulating the position and pressure applied to the TMJ. Specifically, tinnitus sufferers in this group can substantially change their tinnitus by 1) clenching the back teeth tightly; 2) applying resistance to the forehead with a fist as the head pushes forward; 3) opening the mouth to its widest possible point.

In addition to this large number of people who can physically manipulate their tinnitus (thus offering clues for additional useful therapies), we also know that the tympanic membrane (ear drum) is connected to the TMJ by the sphenomandibular ligament—an interesting "coincidence."

Dissections of the ear of corpses have shown this connection, which was once looked upon with skepticism. In 1962, Dr. O. Pinto reported his pioneering work in this area and his discovery of this ligament has been substantiated.

In 1986, Komori duplicated Pinto's work. However, he determined that the anterior malleor ligament was actually two ligaments, the discomalleolar and the sphenomandibular ligament. In 1993, this dissection of the ear and TMJ was done again by Goode and Murikami of Stanford. 'The dissection shows a temporal bone specimen in which the anterior malleolar ligament is demonstrated and then carefully dissected out showing that the ligament in this ear passes all the way from the malleus to the TMJ. Movement of the joint tissue produces a movement of the ligament and malleus. It has been established beyond a doubt that this ligament exists. There is a connection between the ear and the TMJ structures...

In 1992, Chole and Parker did a study on 1,032 patients: 338 had TM disorders and 694 served as two age-matched control groups. Tinnitus and vertigo symptoms were significantly more prevalent in the TMD group than in either of the control groups.

Morgan's conclusion: "We believe we know one of the mechanisms: Appropriate TMJ treatment can help with many ear symptoms, including tinnitus." ("Tinnitus Caused by Temporomandibular Disorder," Douglas Morgan, D.D.S., Proceedings of the Fifth International Tinnitus Seminar, 1995.)

Dr. Douglas Morgan told me in 1993, when I was suffering from severe tinnitus, that TMJ–Disorder is probably regularly caused by stress. Dr. Morgan has researched the relationship between some forms of tinnitus and TMD for over 20 years, and his expert findings bear consideration. If you can alter the quality or sound of your tinnitus through one of the "tests" noted above, I urge you to seek help for TMD from a competent practitioner.

If all TMD is not caused by stress, it is probable that most all cases of TMD are highly correlated to severe stress involvement. Therefore, it is reasonable to assume that those with both tinnitus and TMD are likely to suffer more than those with one or the other — a reminder that multi–modal therapy is very important.

I have spoken with a number of people who have had TMJD corrected either surgically or with *a splint*, and in some cases their tinnitus has reduced or been eliminated. **Craniomandibular Disorder (CMD)** is a term that encompasses most structural problems in the head, including TMJD. *An osteopath can often provide relief not only of head* *pains associated with TMD and CMD by physical manipulation, but can often reduce the volume of your tinnitus by manipulating the head in ways that take pressure off of the TMJ area.* However, your osteopath may not know that he or she actually can do this, so you may have to suggest this option! Many medical doctors listed as osteopaths in the phone book do not actually practice osteopathy. This is understandable, since the insurance company payments for extended osteopathic work are often less than what the doctor receives for seeing patients with sores throats and headaches.

Key Points to Remember in this Chapter

- Tinnitus is experienced in the brain whether it is generated in the ear or brain.
- Because tinnitus is experienced in the brain, you can reduce the volume and distress through therapeutic interventions that cause changes in the brain.
- If your tinnitus is related to hearing loss, it is possible that old brain cells have received new jobs. Your brain cells can be given even newer jobs intentionally through psychotherapy, hypnotherapy, habituation, and medications.
- Tinnitus suffering is an "emotional brain" phenomenon.
- Subjective Idiopathic Tinnitus is a paradoxical memory. This memory is similar to other memories in that it can be forgotten when conscious attention is placed on other stimuli.
- Stress, panic disorder, anxiety, depression and emotional problems (SPADE) have all been correlated to tinnitus, and generally have been correlated to pre-dispose people to tinnitus suffering.
- Tinnitus can be eliminated in some cases, but in general, it can only be eliminated if the sound of the tinnitus becomes irrelevant, meaningless, and unimportant.
- Anti-depressants can eliminate or reduce the volume and suffering of a large percentage of people with tinnitus.
- Benzodiazepines can reduce the volume and distress of tinnitus in a majority of people.
- Tinnitus can be generated in the ear, the head, or both.

- Tinnitus that is "in the head" is generally caused by either blood flow problems, nerve and cellular degeneration, and/or emotional problems such as depression, anxiety, dementia, etc.
- Tinnitus is heard, stored, and evaluated in the media temporal lobe system of the brain, specifically the hippocampal amygdala complex and other parts of the "limbic" system.
- Tinnitus and the Negative Emotions (stress, depression, anxiety, etc.) are hooked together in conditioned response like Pavlov's dogs that were conditioned to salivate when they heard the bell, after the bell sound was paired with food.
- Tinnitus and Negative Emotions must be unhooked at both the conscious and the unconscious level for long-term positive results.
- Extreme volume of tinnitus is associated with suffering, but moderate volume doesn't necessarily cause suffering in any individual person.
- Tinnitus generated from the ear can be caused from many different causes, varying from person to person.
- Caroverine, a drug not yet approved for distribution in the United States, is highly effective in reducing tinnitus volume that is generated in cochlear synaptic tinnitus.
- The TMJ area needs to be relaxed and healthy to help those whose tinnitus is related to TMD.

CHAPTER FOUR
Evaluating Your Emotions & Fine Tuning Treatment Options

The objective we have set for you in this book is to reduce or eliminate: (1) the volume of your tinnitus; and (2) the emotional distress of listening to your tinnitus. This process of emotional and auditory "habituation" normally takes several months, so please be optimistic and allow yourself to be patient.

You will, in all likelihood, reach at least one of the two objectives as you pursue the treatments discussed in this book (and in the related audio programming, should you choose to order the *Tinnitus Reduction Program* available from the back of the book).

It is expected that you will meet your long-term objectives, and many people begin noticing positive results emotionally in a few weeks or less. Significant tinnitus reduction may take several weeks, months, or even years. As you pursue these and other therapies discussed in this book, we suggest you contact the tinnitus association in the country you live in, or write to the association in the country nearest you. There are some tinnitus associations that I have not listed in this book because of their lack of track record. Joining an organization such as the American Tinnitus Association gives you one significant piece of information: You are not alone.

Feelings of loneliness or aloneness can greatly hamper the recovery process. Feeling "connected" has been scientifically shown to speed recovery times in numerous diseases and disorders. With this in mind, let us consider where you are emotionally.

What are Your S.P.A.D.E. Levels?

Numerous tinnitus researchers indicate that depression and/or anxiety exist in all "subjective idiopathic tinnitus" patients.

In the next few pages you can consider your levels of stress and depression. You may have be fortunate and experience comparatively little of either. However, if you have higher stress levels than most people, or experience more bouts with depression, there is good news. What may be the most exciting revelation in the reduction of volume is the significance of emotional distress in tinnitus, and the understanding of *the link between stress, panic disorder, anxiety, depression, and/or emotional disorders with the onset of tinnitus.*

Stress

Stress may be the most overlooked element in the cause of tinnitus. Stress itself may or may not cause tinnitus, but it does help create the psychological environment for onset of tinnitus.

Five thousand people may attend a loud rock concert, and only a few will get permanent tinnitus from the concert. The individuals who experience onset are normally those who are currently experiencing or have in the recent past experienced great stress, depression, panic, anxiety and/or emotional disorders.

It is worth considering how much stress you have been under in the past 18 months. This can be evaluated in a simple but unscientific stress test. The test is offered here and I would urge you to take it now. SPADEs reduce the effectiveness of the immune system and therefore increase the likelihood that tinnitus will onset in individuals scoring high in stress over approximately the previous 18 months. This test is not a diagnostic test, but a test for your self-reference.

Stress may be the most overlooked element in the cause of tinnitus.

(All of the audiocassettes in the *Tinnitus Reduction Program* that focus on hypnotherapeutic interventions as well as relaxation are useful in improving your response to the SPADEs in your environment and within yourself.)

Your Unofficial Stress Evaluation

To determine your total stress points, put a check mark next to each category that applies to you during the previous 18 months. If two events occurred in the same category, make two check marks and double the points. This test was developed many years ago by Holmes and Rahe as a simple and fairly objective scale to determine the amount of stress in an individual's life. It does not include newer forms of stress creators such as computer and internet–related stress, but nonetheless it continues to be a useful self help diagnostic. By adding the numerical values of the various stressful events in your life, you come up with your Total Stress Points.

STRESS EVALUATION

Death of a spouse	100	_____
Divorce (yours)	73	_____
Marital separation (yours)	65	_____
Jail term	63	_____
Death of a close family member	63	_____
Personal injury or illness	53	_____
Marriage (your own)	50	_____
Fired from work	47	_____
Marital reconciliation	45	_____
Retirement	44	_____
Change in family member's health	44	_____
Pregnancy (yours/your wife's)	40	_____
Sexual difficulties	39	_____
Addition to the family	39	_____
Business readjustment	39	_____
Change in financial status	38	_____
Death of a close friend	37	_____
Change to a different line of work	36	_____
Change in number of marital arguments	36	_____
Loan over $10,000	31	_____
Foreclosure of mortgage or loan	30	_____

Change in work responsibilities	29	_____
Son or daughter leaving home	29	_____
Trouble with in–laws	29	_____
Outstanding personal achievement	28	_____
Spouse stops or begins work	26	_____
Starting or finishing school	26	_____
Change in living conditions	25	_____
Revision of personal habits	24	_____
Trouble with boss	23	_____
Change in work hours, conditions	20	_____
Change in residence	20	_____
Change in recreational habits	19	_____
Change in church activities	19	_____
Change in social activities	18	_____
Loan under $10,000	17	_____
Change in sleeping habits	16	_____
Change in number of family gatherings	15	_____
Change in eating habits	15	_____
Vacation	13	_____
Christmas season	12	_____
Minor violation of the law	11	
TOTAL STRESS POINTS		

Approximately one half of all people with stress points over 300 report illnesses during the period under study. Only 10 percent of people with stress points under 200 had illness during the tested period. The more stress points you have, the more likely you are to undergo a significant illness. While you were taking this test, you noticed that many positive events (having a baby, getting married, a better job) are also stressful. An individual's coping capabilities often determine whether or not an he or she will come down with an illness.

Anxiety

Anxiety and stress can be related but, like fraternal twins, they are not identical—just similar. When a person is "anxious," she or he is in a flight or fight state, and the person's senses become heightened. When you are in these kinds of states, what you see, smell, hear, taste, and your sense of touch all become hyper–aware. This instinct is useful for the survival of the self and our species, but not for the reduction of tinnitus. Tinnitus sufferers who experience anxiety are likely to notice their tinnitus exacerbated. Because anxiety is not useful for the tinnitus sufferer, some method of anxiety reduction is suggested, such as the anxiety reducing tape in the *Tinnitus Reduction Program.*

You are already aware that anxiety is a learned behavior, much like a phobia. When events in the environment activate traumatic or fearful memories, a person may experience generalized anxiety or a full blown anxiety "attack." You also are probably aware that anxiety disorders are treatable by methods other than hypnotherapy and self hypnosis.

Depression

There are a number of "types" or "grades" of depression. Depression is often cited as the fertile ground where tinnitus is born. In the early twenty–first century, not only do we live in the most stressful and fast paced time in history, but we also live in a time when more people experience depression than ever before.

When a loved one dies or becomes seriously ill, we often feel helpless and hopeless. Maybe our own personal lives have become so distressing and hopeless that we believe that there is no light at the end of the tunnel. These are common expressions of people who are experiencing depression. It is important to understand this, because once you recognize and verbalize that you are depressed you find it much easier to improve your life.

> Treating depression often reduces tinnitus volume and normally reduces the distress related to tinnitus.

How do you know whether you have or have had depression? Seeing a psychologist or psychiatrist is the best and most efficient way to determine whether you have depression. For the purpose of this program, if you have five or more of symptoms in the following Depression Screening, it is very possible that you have depression, and you are urged to see a mental health professional for your benefit. Remember, tinnitus and depression are correlated in many individuals. Treating depression often reduces tinnitus volume and normally reduces the distress related to tinnitus.

Depression Screening

If you answer "yes" to any phrase. count one point. Count two points for the final phrase. Please remember that this is not an official diagnostic test or an evaluation, and it does not replace a professional opinion. This is offered simply to give you a gauge for your own insight.

DEPRESSION SCREENING

Do you often find yourself in a depressed mood?	_____
Do you have a loss of interest in your usual activities?	_____
Are you experiencing a loss of appetite?	_____
Are you experiencing nights with insomnia?	_____
Are you experiencing psychomotor retardation (slow thought or movement)?	_____
Are you experiencing a loss of energy?	_____
Are you experiencing feelings of worthlessness and/or guilt?	_____
Are you experiencing a diminished ability to think and/or poor concentration?	_____
Have you experienced suicidal thoughts or actions?	
TOTAL	

The last notation, obviously, is a critical one. Anyone who is considering suicide needs to see a competent practitioner for help. **Asking for help is a great sign of strength and courage.**

If you identify only one or two of the top eight "symptoms," you probably are not suffering from what a psychologist would consider depression. If you have three or more "points," you should see a mental health practitioner.

If depression is a contributing factor to your tinnitus, then eliminating the depression will likely reduce the volume and possibly all of the emotional distress related to your tinnitus. Depression is normally not considered a disease, but a sum of its symptoms. It generally involves negative thinking, a pessimistic view of life, neurobiological causes, and a tendency to believe that "bad things happen all the time and there is little that can be done to change that." Overcoming depression, for many people, is a challenging process. With proper help, in all likelihood you will improve and discover a dramatic reduction in the emotional distress created by your tinnitus.

Depression normally begins when a person who is neurobiologically predisposed to depression encounters failure, and interprets that failure in a pessimistic fashion. This is a standard recipe for depressive episodes. The failure validates the negative outlook. When tinnitus begins, the scope widens. An apparently uncontrollable stimulus such as tinnitus often creates another vicious spiral downward. In this case, depression contributes to the tinnitus, and the tinnitus, in turn, makes the depression worse. Depression becomes more and more hopeless, and so on.

Depression does not always bring on tinnitus, and tinnitus doesn't always bring on depression. However, there is a definite relationship between the two in a significant number of tinnitus sufferers. This is one reason that the use of anti-depressant medications not only can improve the quality of life, but also reduce the discomfort of your tinnitus. One study revealed that:

- people with tinnitus are far more likely than others to have experienced a virtual life–long depression.
- 78 percent of individuals with tinnitus have had a prevalence of lifetime depression, compared to only 21 percent of a control group.
- 60 percent of tinnitus sufferers, apparently, were experiencing depression at the time of the study, compared to 7 percent of those in a control group.
- 48 percent of individuals with tinnitus had suffered at least one major depression in the past, compared to 14 percent of a control group.

All of these numbers highlight the powerful link between depression and tinnitus. The same study also showed that those people who are disabled by tinnitus can often be helped back to normal life by treating the depression and its causes.

Those who do not seek help may have many problems directly or indirectly caused by the combination of depression and tinnitus. These include problems with cognitive function, physical appearance, body deterioration, sexual function, contact with family and friends, and assertive behavior. **Individuals with both depression and tinnitus also suffer about three times as many other physical ailments than do control groups.**

A key component of depression that will need to be changed first is that of rumination. Constantly and repetitiously mulling over a problem such as tinnitus will make the tinnitus worse. Getting involved in fun activities, productive projects, and the loves of life will immediately improve the individual's state of mind. If you are experiencing depression or feelings of helplessness, read Dr. Martin Seligman's brilliant book,

Learned Optimism, for ways to cope with depression without the use of drugs. This book is not a typical self help book. It is based on solid scientific research that can be critical to helping you on your road to quieter days.

Panic Attacks

Panic disorder is another common pre-disposing condition of tinnitus. **Over half of all individuals suffering from panic disorder suffered with tinnitus,** according to results of a recent study on various anxiety–related difficulties such as panic attacks—generally anxiety disorder and social phobia

With 48 individuals in the study, the following symptoms were noted in at least half of the panic attack sufferers:

1) Palpitations	43
2) Fatigue	35
3) Chest Pain	33
4) Muscle tension	33
5) Persisting nervousness	32
6) Restlessness	31
7) Sweating/flushing	28
8) Trembling/shaking	28
9) **Tinnitus**	**27**
10) Lightheadedness	25

In other words, *56 percent of the people in this study with panic disorder also had tinnitus.* Very few studies have been done in the area of establishing a link between panic disorder and tinnitus; however, this particular study strongly suggests such a link.

The good news is that panic disorder, like stress, anxiety and depression is treatable, and can be largely eliminated. The two most effective interventions for panic disorder are Benzodiazepines (Xanax, Ativan, Valium, etc.), some anti-depressants, and hypnotherapy. The self-hypnosis tapes in the *Tinnitus Reduction Program* will be very useful in addressing both tinnitus and panic symptoms.

Alcohol Dependence

I was somewhat surprised to read a recent study revealing that **38 percent of current tinnitus sufferers were shown to have a past dependence on alcohol**—about three times as high as the control group norm. Alcoholism and addiction to alcohol are treatable, and also another contributing cause of tinnitus that can be reduced through self hypnosis and hypnotherapy.

Other studies have shown that tinnitus is exacerbated by alcohol. It is generally recommended that individuals suffering from tinnitus should greatly reduce or eliminate alcohol intake if they wish to improve. Another recent study showed that, while it is true that alcohol exacerbates tinnitus in about one—fourth of individuals, it is also true that about one in five gains relief from tinnitus with very moderate alcohol intake.

Personality Characteristics of Tinnitus Sufferers

Recent studies reveal that certain personality traits have been correlated to individuals who later develop tinnitus. To increase the likelihood of your success in tinnitus reduction, you want to learn how people may perceive some tinnitus sufferers. This determines how others respond to you in day to day life, thus affecting the way you feel. It is also useful to gain personal insights into how you behave and the stress that your state of mind can cause you. Several traits have been positively correlated to the tinnitus sufferer. In my practice I have found the average tinnitus sufferer to be of above average IQ, but below average in areas of emotional coping, and for good reason. This section of the book will touch on a few of the key traits tinnitus literature correlates to tinnitus sufferers. Addressing these traits head on may expedite your healing process.

The first trait that is evident in research is the characteristic of *introspection*. The characteristic of introspection can be a marvelous personality trait for individuals to adopt. However, because of the nature of introspection, the intrusiveness of tinnitus gets in the way of the peace of mind highly introspective people crave, and can actually cause these individuals to become unkind, incommunicative or even hostile.

Are you a *perfectionist*? So are many other sufferers of tinnitus. What can you do to reduce your need to be perfect while still allowing yourself excellence?

There is a body of research that reveals the tinnitus sufferer often considers himself a *victim*. Although this is certainly true to a degree, it is far more useful to perceive tinnitus as something that will soon be under control of the individual. A victim is helpless. A person in control can find constructive choices and methods to solve problems. No one goes seeking tinnitus. Unfortunately, lifestyles and lifestyle choices often trigger tinnitus. Because of the interrelationship of personality, neurological difficulties, TMD, audiological deficiencies, and other difficulties, any person experiencing tinnitus may feel that tinnitus is a challenge of enormous height.

That is why it takes a team of professionals and a multi-modal approach to help reduce tinnitus volume and distress. No one echoes this sentiment more than Dr. Robert Sweetow of the University of California, San Francisco.

> *Not all clinicians feel equipped to provide the types of interventions discussed [in this paper]. In addition, direct counseling from a trained psychologist or psychiatrist may be in order. Tinnitus patients have been described as rigid, desperate, obsessive and neurotic. Many present with additional problems contributing to tinnitus distress (i.e., divorce, lack of money, dissatisfaction with their occupations. Some have a history of clinical depression). A team that has been established at UCSF includes **audiologists, otologists, temporomandibular–joint specialists, psychologists, psychiatrists, physical therapists, biofeedback specialists, pharmacologists, and nutritionists**.*
>
> "The Evolution of Cognitive-Behavioral Therapy as an Approach to Tinnitus Patient Management," Robert Sweetow, Ph.D. *International Journal of Tinnitus*, 1995.

Tinnitus patients, as a whole, tend to feel more sensitive about personal matters. They also tend to have feelings of persecution more so than control groups. Can you identify with these characteristics? If you experience these feelings and exhibit these traits, you have an edge in the arena of awareness.

It is a good sign that you are aware of your personality. This makes constructing new behaviors a much simpler process.

Personality traits such as those mentioned above, can not only lead to tinnitus, but once the tinnitus has started, can act as a causal factor in creating the feedback loops discussed throughout this book. It is very reasonable that a person who suddenly has a siren in his head is going to feel persecuted, and none of the normal things the person does to cope with pain seem to help tinnitus. This feeling of helplessness is completely understandable. The good news is that the feeling of helplessness can be short lived once you take steps toward improvement.

> Awareness of your personality makes constructing new behaviors a much simpler process.

Ruling out Dangerous Causes Before Treatment

It seems wise to me that anyone with persistent tinnitus would seriously consider being examined through an MRI, or at the very least a CT scan. MRI (multi-resonance imaging) is safe for most people and, although it is a noisy process, it is certainly useful in ruling out tumors, cysts, or other growths in the head that may cause tinnitus. In these cases the growths can be life–threatening, although rarely cancerous in nature. It seems prudent always to be certain your life is in no danger before beginning any medical treatment.

In my personal practice, I have had two female clients who requested (and did not receive) MRIs from their medical doctors, and later were deafened when they had to have large tumors surgically removed from the eighth nerve. Both women were wise enough to ask for the precaution of an MRI, only to be turned down and given a life of unilateral deafness. In neither case did the tinnitus subside after surgery. Had they been given MRIs, the tumors would have been discovered while they were small, and, in all likelihood, the tumors would have been removed and the auditory nerve saved. *Always get an MRI or CT scan.*

CHAPTER FIVE
Effective Treatment Methods for Tinnitus Reduction

Throughout this book numerous treatments for tinnitus while we discussed have been discussed along with causes. In this section, I want to address important and effective therapeutic interventions to put you on the road to greater peace of mind.

Research has shown that there are a few key modalities for tinnitus reduction, and numerous others that work on occasion. **Medication, masking, habituation,** and **hypnotherapy** are among the most effective methods for treating tinnitus. Biofeedback and massage therapy have been shown to be helpful as well, though we will not discuss them in great detail here. Each of the most effective treatment modalities will now be discussed at some length.

Masking & Tinnitus Habituation Therapy

Most, but not all people who suffer from tinnitus gain benefit through masking and/or habituation.

- **Masking,** a common method of dealing with tinnitus, is the "covering" of the noise that is in the head or ears with noise that is external to the head and ears.

- **Tinnitus Habituation Therapy** is the process of adding broad band white noise in small increments to "re-train the auditory pathways," so that the sound of the tinnitus no longer creates a negative emotional response. Specifically, the tinnitus sufferer wears a "walkman" or specially made "white noise generators" every day, all the time. The noise produced by the external source creates a smaller distinction between a neutral stimulus and the tinnitus.

When I was travelling on my own road to peace I wore a walkman to bed and all day long, including during my session time with clients. It was an inconvenience, but the process was effective in helping the habituation process. Many others have successfully utilized habituation.

> Masking is the "covering" of the noise that is in the head or ears with noise that is external to the head and ears.

Unfortunately, masking and habituation do not work with profoundly deaf people, nor with individuals who have severe hearing loss. These methods are very slow for people with severe hyperacusis. For those who do have most of their hearing, masking and habituation are interesting options.

One common method of masking is the use of a hearing aid/tinnitus masker. Essentially, a hearing aid is worn in the ear(s) that has tinnitus, and a new sound is generated by the masker to cover the tinnitus. In the habituation process the sound is not turned up to cover the sound, but is set just below the threshold of the tinnitus. This creates a "new" sound for the brain to "find."

Tinnitus maskers that are worn as hearing aids are comfortable to wear, and the white noise is far more pleasant than that of the tinnitus. The drawback to tinnitus maskers is that you must wear them all of the time. Most tinnitus maskers cost about $700 to $1,500 per ear. Batteries will cost about $100, and must be replaced regularly.

Other types of tinnitus maskers are not worn, but are used by the bedside or in the office.

> Tinnitus Habituation Therapy is the process of adding broad-band white noise in small increments to "re-train the auditory pathways," so that the sound of the tinnitus no longer creates a negative emotional response.

Commonly, these are white noise generators that can mask or habituate the sound of the tinnitus as well. Some machines produce many tones, so that the user can select a band that covers her tinnitus. Other machines produce sounds that emulate rain fall, ocean waves, and other pleasant environmental sounds. These machines are inexpensive and remarkably valuable to the sufferer of tinnitus.

I used a personal stereo with headphones as a method of both habituating and masking my tinnitus for two reasons. First, the cost was minimal, and environmental and classical music audiocassettes were a superior option for me when contrasted to the static sound of white noise. Secondly, I believe that listening to sounds to which I already had a positive emotional response created speedier habituation than I might have attained with neutral or slightly negative static/white noise sounds.

Some people find that de-tuning their radio to a place in between FM stations, with static, is very helpful in masking tinnitus. Others select audio cassettes that cover the tinnitus or help habituate it. Classical music and new age music tapes have proven effective in using personal stereos for relief.

I highly recommend the use of "habituators" or a "walkman." If you do not decide in favor of this therapeutic option, it is a very good idea to constantly have background noise "on" so that you experience less stress due to tinnitus, on a daily basis. Background noise makes the tinnitus less detectable in almost all clients I have worked with.

Some of my clients have followed in my footsteps and decided to wear and listen to their walkman all night with headphones. Having comfortable earphones or "dots" that actually fit into the ear is critical to sleeping with ease.

Tinnitus Habituation Therapy

Dr. Pawel Jastreboff has pioneered research in the tinnitus habituation process at the University of Maryland. I have attempted to describe an adaptation of Dr. Jastreboff's strategy for tinnitus habituation on the next page. I would recommend contacting Dr. Jastreboff's office for further information about THT. His research in the field is widely respected, and has been critical in developing therapeutic interventions that are helping thousands of people worldwide. Please consult your audiologist for additional information, and be certain to consult your medical practitioner before beginning any treatment for tinnitus.

Self-Help Program for Habituation

1) Once it is determined, through testing, that there is no major medical problem causing tinnitus, tinnitus habituation therapy can be attempted with tinnitus white noise generators. Any manufacturer is probably as good as another.

2) It is very important for the individual to accept the understanding that tinnitus is similar to chronic pain: It is annoying but it is not life threatening. Tinnitus can be eliminated, or at least reduced.

3) It takes time to make progress in habituation therapy. Patience is important. Most people do not experience instant results in habituation therapy.

4) A tinnitus "masker" or white noise generator should be used during all waking hours.

5) When beginning your self help therapy, you should use a very soft level of white noise. Use a level that you can barely hear in each ear.

6) Each week turn up the volume of the generators just a bit.

7) Stop turning up the volume when it is no longer quiet, but not extremely loud.
8) If the noise level ever increases the tinnitus of the individual, reduce the volume of the generator.
9) Do not increase the volume of the generator over that of the tinnitus.

This self help program for habituation is based on my work with clients and the published papers of Pawel Jastreboff, R. R. Coles, Jean Baskill, Jonathon Hazel, and Jacqueline Sheldrake. My simple outline is not necessarily endorsed by the researchers in any way. My retraining therapy model is simply one that can be used by an individual while waiting what may be years to see one of the professionals in the habituation field. If you are fortunate, this self help therapy will succeed before you ever see one of the leaders in the profession.

The cause of tinnitus is normally not important when using habituation. Habituation is completely safe and poses no side effects. At the University of Maryland, over an 18–month period, the following results were published:

> *84 percent have significant improvement in both decreased annoyance of the tinnitus and definite habituation to its perception...*
> "Tinnitus Habituation Therapy: The University of Maryland Tinnitus and Hyperacusis Center Experience," Douglas Mattox, M.D., Pawel Jastreboff, Ph.D., William Gray, M.D., *International Journal of Tinnitus*, 1997.

Effective Medication for Tinnitus Reduction

Masking and habituation procedures are limited modalities of treatments, of course. Medication may be the best option for many individuals. Medications that tend to improve tinnitus fall into three major categories. They work fairly quickly (usually tinnitus and distress levels ease in fewer than three months) and they are safe. However, most people experience some kind of side effects from using these medications. Side effects tend to be minor when compared to suicidal thoughts or severe depression, anxiety, and stress related to tinnitus distress. Each individual will be able to carefully evaluate and weigh side effects in contrast to tinnitus suffering, as time goes on. Side effects tend to occur rapidly (within a few days), whereas the benefit from the medications tend to occur in 4 to 8 weeks. Patience is the key.

Anti–anxiety	Xanax, Ativan, Valium, Serax, etc.
Anti–depressant	Zoloft, Pamelor, Effextor, Paxil, Serzone, etc.
Anti–convulsant	Tegretol, Primidone, Klonopin, etc.

Medications normally begin to reduce tinnitus far more quickly than do masking and habituation. A medication such as Xanax may begin to reduce tinnitus volume and distress in as little as 8 weeks, and normally in less than 12 weeks.

Anti-anxiety

The most common medications used to reduce tinnitus are benzodiazepines. Benzodiazepines and other anti-anxiety medications selectively reduce anxiety in the central nervous system. Because of the phenomenon of "hyper-awareness," it is often beneficial to reduce excitatory activity in the brain and the central nervous system. Anti-anxiety medications often succeed in reducing the volume and stress of tinnitus.

Xanax, (generic: alprazolam) is a commonly prescribed drug for tinnitus sufferers. In a recent double blind placebo study, **76 percent of individuals using Xanax experienced over 40 percent reduction of volume in their tinnitus.** Unfortunately, Xanax does not normally completely eliminate tinnitus. It does succeed in volume and stress reduction for most people, however.

Some people have discovered side effects of Xanax that make it difficult to use. Some of these common side effects (more than one in 20 people may be affected) include blurred vision, change in sex drive, constipation, drowsiness, dry mouth, fatigue, and headache.

It should be noted that when Xanax is used for tinnitus, it is normally prescribed in very small doses. Generally medical doctors will begin a prescription at .25 mg per dose, three times daily. Over a period of two or three weeks they will increase the dose to .5 mg per dose three times daily. Once this level is maintained for 4 to 10 weeks, the patient can expect reduction and relief to begin, if it is going to.

When eliminating Xanax as a treatment modality, it is best to gradually reduce dosages. Your doctor will explain to you the best reduction program for you. *Never simply stop taking Xanax or any benzodiazepine.* Xanax can be habituating (similar to addiction) in some, but certainly not all, people.

Medications in this class of drugs that have fared best are **Serax** and **Klonopin.** One controlled study by Dr. Abraham

Shulman reported that Serax reduced tinnitus volume in 52 percent of patients. Klonopin was effective in 69 percent (virtually identical to the Xanax results).

Other medications in this family of drugs that seem to be useful in treating tinnitus include Ativan, Traxene, and Valium.

Anti-convulsant

Anti-convulsants have been prescribed for tinnitus for many years. Normally these medications are used to prevent seizures, but because of action of these medications within the brain, large numbers of people with tinnitus have reported improvement from their use. Anti-convulsants work by selectively reducing excessive stimulation in the brain. Interestingly, they can be effective in reducing tinnitus volume and provide relief, as well. **Tegretol,** or **Klonopin** are frequently prescribed for tinnitus sufferers. This family of drugs is among the original pharmacological interventions for tinnitus sufferers. It is interesting to note that about 80 percent of people who have nearly all of their tinnitus eliminated from lidocaine infusions also experience very significant volume reduction with Tegretol.

Who should use Tegretol, or the other anti-epileptic/convulsants? People whose tinnitus is central (not one side or the other), disabling in nature, and have failed at Tinnitus Habituation Therapy would be candidates. People whose tinnitus fluctuates in volume from day to day seem to benefit more from Tegretol than those with other tinnitus experiences.

Most medical doctors will start a patient with 100mg. of Tegretol per day and slowly work up to 500 to 2,000 mg. per day. The smallest dosage that reduces volume would be optimal. There are side effects to Tegretol, which can be significant deterrents for some people. Talk to your medical practitioner.

One study with Primidone reported 27 percent experienced almost complete tinnitus elimination. Another 59 percent reported significant relief (20 to 80 percent volume reduction).

Anti-depressant

It may surprise you to know that in selected tinnitus patients, with time, anti-depressants can virtually eliminate tinnitus. There are a number of anti-depressants, and not all work equally as well in all tinnitus sufferers for volume reduction, so some trial and error experimentation may be necessary.

Two types of anti-depressants that have worked well are the tricyclics and the SSRIs. Tricyclic anti-depressants block uptake of norepinephrine and/or serotonin into the pre-synaptic neuron, making more neurotransmitter available in the synapse. Tricyclic antidepressants that have been tested for tinnitus reduction include **Pamelor** (generic name: nortryptiline) and **Elavil** (amitryptiline). Where **Pamelor has shown excellent results in reducing tinnitus volume,** it is interesting to note that Elavil, while also helpful sometimes, actually induces tinnitus in some people. Pamelor and Elavil, coincidentally, also help individuals with panic, insomnia, and severe depression. These medications are often prescribed for individuals with migraines and chronic pain. Common side effects (more than 5 percent) include dry mouth, blurred vision, dizziness, weight gain, sedation, and arousal.

The SSRIs (selective serotonin re-uptake inhibitors) include **Paxil, Zoloft, Prozac,** and **Luvox.** In simple language, these drugs keep serotonin "working" in the brain, improving the mood of the patient and reducing depression levels.

Vast amounts of media coverage regarding these medications and other similar ones have created polarized views that are often not accurate. One fact is certain. Many people credit anti-depressant medications for the major volume reduction in tinnitus they have experienced. (I successfully used Zoloft. It reduced about 40 percent of the noise experienced.)

Serotonin is the oldest neurotransmitter to have been found on the evolutionary chain, having been witnessed even in snails.

> *The many connections of serotonin–containing
> neurons allow this neurotransmitter to be involved in
> the regulation of numerous basic psychobiological
> functions including appetite, sexual interest, sleep,
> pain perception, bodily rhythms, mood and thought.
> Serotonin also appears to play a significant role in
> regulation of impulsivity and the unpremeditated kind
> of aggression that arises abruptly in response to
> frustration. Serotonin often works in the opposite
> direction of norepinephrine, transmitting soothing
> signals of calm and rest that stabilize emotional
> responses.*
> Steven Dubovsky, M.D., *Mind-Body Deceptions,*
> Norton Publishing, 1997.

It is for this reason that I believe anti-depressants are as effective as they are in reducing tinnitus volume and distress. When serotonin is allowed to do its job in the brain, it reduces negative responses to stimuli, as noted above. I believe this to also include the negative response to tinnitus that tinnitus sufferers experience.

> ...*all anti-depressant medications are equally effective in treating depression, and, with the exception of bupropion (Wellbutrin), all antidepressants seem to be useful for different forms of anxiety as well as for depression. Differences in side effects profiles help physicians choose one antidepressant over another for a specific patient. For example, because serotonin reduces aggressive outbursts, a serotonin reuptake inhibitor may be useful for depressed people with high levels of irritability, while the sedating effects of a medication like imipramine or one of the newer antidepressants like nefazodone (Serzone) makes these antidepressants desirable for the treatment of depressed people who cannot fall asleep. On the other hand, tricyclic antidepressants tend to have cardiac effects that are problematic for patients with heart block, while the serotonin reuptake inhibitors can make migraine headaches worse.*
> Dubovsky, 1997.

SSRIs are also commonly prescribed for obsessive compulsive disorder, post traumatic stress disorder, and bulimia. Common side effects for the SSRIs include jitteriness, sexual dysfunction, headache, and gastrointestinal distress.

Allow six to eight weeks for antidepressants to take effect. Some side effects reduce in a few days. Carefully consult with your medical doctor.

Note: As with anti-anxiety and anti-convulsant medications, when discontinuing the use of these medications, it is important to stop gradually and slowly and keep your medical doctor informed of your withdrawing process. A number of other new antidepressant medications are likely to be effective in helping the tinnitus sufferer. Ask your doctor for further advice.

Over–the–Counter Remedies

Over–the–counter remedies are normally useless for tinnitus, with the exception of an herb called **ginkgo biloba**. Ginkgo is available in most health food stores. Studies to date about ginkgo tend to be mixed as far as its usefulness in reducing the volume of tinnitus. Ginkgo may be effective in about one third of tinnitus sufferers because it tends to improve vascular functioning. It acts as a vasodilator, widening blood vessels and improving blood flow. Ginkgo has also been shown to have positive effects for Alzheimer's patients, which leads one to be optimistic about its further use for tinnitus as well. It is likely that ginkgo is most effective for people with central tinnitus.

It is possible that **St. John's Wort,** an herb that acts like an MAO Inhibitor for depression, may help in tinnitus distress reduction. It is also possible that the herb **kava kava** may help reduce anxiety. If the claims made by the manufacturers and proponents of these herbs are true, studies could well be done to test their effectiveness in treating tinnitus.

There are no other herb or over-the-counter remedies, or homeopathic remedies that have been shown to have efficacy in treating tinnitus at this time.

You now have a fundamental understanding of tinnitus and the medications that are likely to help you. Speak with your health professional, and bring this book along for your physician to look at so she or he understands that you are seriously ready to begin your healing process.

Hypnotherapy for Tinnitus Reduction

Recent research reveals that the results of well–constructed self hypnosis programs nearly equal the results of Tinnitus Retraining Therapy and Xanax for volume and distress reduction. In fact, almost everyone should benefit from reduced distress after utilizing self-hypnosis cassettes designed for tinnitus sufferers for 90 days or more. A well–trained, experienced hypnotherapist is likely to be help you more than an audiocassette program.

It has always been an embarrassment to me that it took me quite some time to discover that tinnitus could really be reduced through hypnosis. In fact, when my tinnitus was firing off at 75+ dB, I never dreamed hypnotherapy could be effective for volume reduction. Much to the surprise of this clinical hypnotherapist, what I found through personal experience, and then research, then working with hundreds of clients, was that even when hypnotherapy does not eventually eliminate tinnitus, it normally reduces the volume, the stress, and negative emotions surrounding tinnitus. In fact, one recent study showed that 73 percent of individuals taking part in a study on the efficacy of hypnosis in tinnitus reduction, succeeded in doing just that. Other studies using hypnosis for tinnitus reduction **report between 50 and 76 percent of subjects reducing volume and distress in their tinnitus.**

Astonishing numbers! Some of these studies are outlined in the abstracts in the back of this book.

Why don't more people pursue such a successful therapy? It would seem that there is a perception of hypnosis that is negative in the minds of many. Generally, I believe this is attributable to the media's common

> Studies using hypnosis for tinnitus reduction report between 50 and 76 percent of subjects reducing volume and distress in their tinnitus.

portrayal of hypnotists. People seem to relate hypnosis to the surrender of will to another person; that is, until they actually participate in hypnotherapy and learn self-hypnosis!

Hypnosis is an old word that once meant sleep, another common misperception. When a person is in a state of hypnosis he or she is often actually in a state that is the exact opposite state of sleep! The generic term hypnosis more accurately describes a state of *heightened awareness* and *focused concentration*. This specific state is scientifically measurable by instruments, and is known as "the alpha state." (Measured by an EEG, this is 8–12 Hz.) Recent studies have shown this state of mind to be superior for learning, recall of memory, and training the mind to overcome the bad "programming" of the past, including tinnitus. Other states of mind may be included under the broad term hypnosis that are not "alpha states."

Countless studies have shown that people who suffer from tinnitus tend to have more somatics than are experienced by the population as a whole. In general, people who suffer from tinnitus suffered from either depression or stress related anxiety before the onset of the noise. This fact, in part, explains the efficacy of hypnosis in the relief of tinnitus. For many decades it has been known that hypnosis reduces stress, anxiety, and phobias. We are learning that hypnotherapy is effective in the treatment of depression, and now, in the treatment of tinnitus.

When a person has tinnitus or any illness, there are emotional clusters of feelings attached to the illness within the neurology of the individual. In psychology, these are known as **state dependent memories.** These memories are powerful because of the emotional attachment to them. With tinnitus, the emotions can run the gamut from anger to anxiety, from distress to depression.

The hypnotherapist's job is two–fold. She or he must defuse the emotional charge from the associations so that the person has a better opportunity for healing. Once the emotional clusters have been removed, the therapist then helps the client's unconscious mind focus on stimuli other than the noise.

Some hypnotherapists will recommend the use of an audio tape after the initial session with the therapist. Generally this tape will allow the individual to use self hypnosis on a daily basis at no additional cost. This form of hypnotherapy has been studied on several occasions with results of improvement ranging from about two–thirds to three–quarters. **Hypnotherapy, therefore, has a demonstrated success rate comparable to auditory habituation and benzodiazepines. Unfortunately there are less than a dozen hypnotherapists in the United States with expertise in working with tinnitus sufferers.**

It's important to note that hypnosis is 100 percent safe for the client, with one caveat. **Hypnosis should not be used until pathology has been determined by a medical doctor.** It would be foolish to silence the noise of tinnitus that was caused by a tumor.

One continuing problem is that fewer than 40 hypnotherapists in the United States have learned how to work with clients experiencing severe tinnitus. For assistance in finding a practitioner, or to work with the author of this program, you can call toll free 1-888-707-1896. Outside of the United States you can call 1-612-707-1898.

Hypnotherapy has a demonstrated success rate comparable to auditory habituation and benzodiazepines.

What Can You Expect in a Hypnotherapy Session?

Each hypnotherapist has a slightly different style, much like a psychologist would. However there are a few hypnotherapeutic models that are common in reducing tinnitus volume and other somatics.

Most hypnotherapists are really skilled only in helping their clients relax. Relaxation is an important element in the healing process of any disorder or disease. Relaxation is not to be sold short, but, in the case of tinnitus and hyperacusis, we need to relax *and* also address the specific feedback loops that are persisting within the mind/brain of the tinnitus sufferer. This is why it is so difficult to find a hypnotherapist skilled in tinnitus therapy. Even medical practitioners who perform hypnosis generally have little knowledge of advanced hypnotic techniques. Here are some of the techniques with which you want your practitioner to have years of skill and experience. You can make specific inquiries of practitioners you will interview to be on your healing team.

Regression Therapy

Regression therapy is one form of hypnotherapy. In regression therapy, the client is regressed to a time before the onset of the tinnitus to discover the trigger of the noise, if it is unknown. Approximately half of all individuals do not know how their tinnitus onset. This will come out in therapy, in most cases. Generally speaking, from this point the therapist can help the client in a couple of ways.

The therapist may have the client simply re-experience onset over and over until the emotional impact becomes boring or even amusing to the client. This is an effective form of systematic desensitization that re-educates the amygdala, so it no longer sends out the flight–or–fight survival responses into the brain and body.

The other traditional methodology is to bring the onset to the client's conscious awareness so the client can make a cognitive decision about how he should feel about tinnitus. Often the tinnitus will reduce in volume at this point.

Ego State Therapy

Ego State Therapy (also known as Parts Therapy) is another form of hypnotherapy that is used for tinnitus. Generally speaking, hypnotherapists work under the assumption that the unconscious mind always does what it thinks is best for the survival of the individual. There are parts of the unconscious that regulate heartbeat, breathing, and blood flow, among all the other neurological functions of the body. All of these can be altered in hypnosis by working with the unconscious.

In parts therapy, we discover what "part" of the mind (not to be confused with the term "brain.") is maintaining the noise of tinnitus, and we negotiate with that part to tell us why the noise is being maintained. Quite often it comes up in therapy that the noise is a signal to the conscious mind. Often it is a message to begin to listen to the self or others, or to make a major life change, frequently work–related. When the "part" is satisfied that the message can get through without the noise, the part often happily gives up its job, and rests. Parts therapy can be miraculous in nature. This author has personally participated in remarkable sessions using parts therapy.

Suggestive Therapy

Suggestive therapy is hypnotherapy that works by suggestion. It is the quickest form of hypnosis, generally working via post-hypnotic suggestion. In this form of therapy, the therapist does not look for causes or parts. Here, the therapist is only concerned with future events and offers the unconscious suggestions. For example:

> *And upon returning to your wide aware state of mind, you will notice the noise that was so distracting earlier today will now be faint, and will signal to you to lead a more peaceful life and spend more time relaxing...*

An excellent therapist will incorporate all three of these general therapies, in addition to teaching the client self-hypnosis for relaxation. Self-hypnosis can be used to relax and experience calmer states of mind without the need of seeing the therapist for relaxation techniques again.

Frequently, it will be necessary and desirable to have a follow up session with a hypnotherapist. A good hypnotherapist will usually charge substantially less for a follow up session, and will work with the client to make sure the work previously done is, indeed, working.

Hypnotherapy is not a "cure" for most cases of severe tinnitus. Hypnosis is an extremely affordable and very helpful therapy for reducing or eliminating the noise and/or the emotional impact of tinnitus. Depending on the cause of the tinnitus and the psychological status of the individual, hypnosis will generally surprise the client with its seemingly amazing results.

Searching for a competent hypnotherapist can be a challenge on your own. When you do contact a hypnotherapist, psychotherapist, or practitioner of any kind, find out how many people with tinnitus they have worked with. Ask if they experience tinnitus themselves. If they claim a great deal of experience in working with people with tinnitus, then they should easily be able to explain to you what you are experiencing long before you get to their office. **Beware of practitioners who claim to have worked with many clients or patients with tinnitus but know little about tinnitus.**

Experienced practitioners who claim to work with tinnitus patients should know at least most of what is in this book. Network 3000 Publishing sells an audio and video program to medical and mental health practitioners that carefully explains how to work with clients experiencing severe tinnitus. You can demand they get at least the basics before using you as their first guinea pig. Recommend the program to your medical professional. Call 1-888-707-1896 to order the video program today.

Waiting for the Noise Reduction: The Waiting Game

It is possible that you will decide to pursue masking or Tinnitus Retraining Therapy (auditory habituation) to reduce your tinnitus. Most masking or habituation programs make no promises, but normally have excellent results after one to two years. Hypnotherapy can have very rapid results, but the success is very much variable from practitioner to practitioner. Some people hear significant results in the reduction of volume in 6 to 12 weeks. Others may not see results for one year or more. Pharmaceuticals will often produce excellent results in fewer than three months. Of course there are challenges involved in using various medications. Some people experience side effects to medication. Others may not get the results they had hoped for.

All of these possible time frames and scenarios demand one thing on the part of the tinnitus listener. There is the request for an "unfair patience." We are given no promise of dates and times of reduction in any scenario involved. In response to this request, the next section was written.

It can be a very difficult time, waiting for improvement. There can be days that seem to unforgivably test our stamina, emotional strength, and outlook on life. Here are some useful ideas that you can use immediately in the meantime. You can turn your "meantime" into a simple and occasionally challenging waiting time.

Focus of Attention...

You may have been told that you should, "just ignore your tinnitus." *This is not possible!*

Please ignore the imagined picture you have in your mind of President Bush. Ignore it now. Ignore it. You see, you cannot ignore something that you are trying to ignore.

What you *can* do is create an external focus of attention. Remember the last time you were fascinated by a book or entranced in an excellent speech? You were externally focused. In psychology, this is what is known as a *flow state.* When you are completely in a flow state, you cannot hear your tinnitus, regardless of its volume. Now this may seem difficult to believe, but it is true.

> You may have been told that you should, "just ignore your tinnitus." This is not possible. You cannot ignore something that you are trying to ignore.

It has been scientifically proven that the conscious mind can only focus on about 126 tiny bits of information each second. Everything else that is in our environment (which amounts to over one million bits of information per second being recorded in the unconscious mind!) still enters into our mind, but it is not in our conscious awareness. When you are thoroughly wrapped up in something that is exciting or enticing to you, your tinnitus is not important enough to the brain to be decoded. As long as the reticular activating system has decided to focus on one set of stimuli, you will not hear the noise in the circuitry of the brain.

You can take full advantage of these facts of your neurological wiring by participating in the most enjoyable activities you know. Your conscious mind will then be directed toward external activity that creates a flow state for you. Unfortunately, activities that demand a great deal of internal processing will normally not be quite as useful for creating a focus of your attention. For example, chess is a game that creates flow states in people who enjoy playing chess, but because the game is largely played inside of the mind, it is more difficult to achieve quiet than in games such as tennis, baseball, basketball, and volleyball, and in hobbies that mostly happen "outside."

Prelude to Auditory Habituation

Many people have discovered that being in a very quiet room and being in a very loud room accomplish the same thing for their tinnitus: Both make the noise go up in volume. The noise increases in a quiet room because more attention units are focused onto the noise itself. This creates a perception of increased volume in the mind of the tinnitus listener.

In a loud room, two key elements cause the volume to increase. First, is the contrast principle. After leaving a loud room we are hyper–aware of noise in our heads. There is a great contrast between the loud environment and the quieter environment. Then there is the simple fact of noise–induced tinnitus. High decibel noises can cause and/or exacerbate tinnitus.

Therefore, it would be prudent to avoid silent and noisy environments. It is best to offer yourself a free prelude to the auditory habituation process. Keep some noise in "the background" in every environment possible. Unless you are profoundly deaf, you can play soft classical musical music, environmental tapes, new age cassettes, or simply use the radio or television to create background noise for your listening. If you do not do this, your brain will normally seek out the original unwelcome tinnitus.

If you are profoundly deaf, then you have an additional challenge. For the deaf, it is actually best to create two different foci. One will be complete focused attention on the tinnitus. Literally meditate on the noise itself for 10 to 15 minutes every day. This will be challenging at first for most tinnitus listeners. However, you will be excited to discover the difference you experience when you participate in externally focused events when you are in a flow state. Because profound deafness robs the individual of external

> Tinnitus as a signal to care for our health, happiness, and those we love is a useful point of view to adopt.

auditory stimuli, you should be aware that the emotional interpretation we place on the tinnitus is very important. It is not necessary to try to convince yourself to "fall in love" with the noise, but it is useful to use the noise as a signal. Many of my clients learn to use tinnitus as a signal to discover *who* they should be "listening to." Other clients learn to use their tinnitus as a message to themselves to care for themselves and others more. Even the profoundly deaf need to listen—pay attention—to themselves and others.

Tinnitus as a signal to care for our health, happiness, and those we love is a useful point of view to adopt. By considering this possibility we do not hate the noises we hear, but emotionally accept them. Emotional restructuring is just as important as auditory habituation isn't it? The hypnotherapy audiocassettes in the Tinnitus Reduction Program will help address emotional issues because they work at the unconscious level, much as a professional hypnotherapist does.

Tinnitus Associations

While pursuing your best course of treatment, there are several resources you will want to utilize to make your time with this noise as easy as possible.

The American Tinnitus Association (ATA), an organization based in Oregon, has helped thousands of tinnitus sufferers with their publication, *Tinnitus Today,* and with a useful medical referral service. As you may have discovered, the medical community is often unaware of how best to treat tinnitus. The ATA has helped make strides for tinnitus listeners by creating a database of providers across the country. Some medical and mental health providers in their database are worth their weight in gold. Others have done more damage than for clients I have worked with.

American Tinnitus Association
PO Box 5
Portland, Oregon 97207-0005
phone 503-248-9985

fax 503-248-0024
toll free phone (within US) 800-634-8978
website www.ata.org
email tinnitus@ata.org

Founded in 1971, the ATA has a staff of helpful people who may be able to steer you in the right direction. They ask for a donation of about $25 per year for becoming a member. Members receive a publication, *Tinnitus Today* quarterly that often contains useful articles. I personally recommend you purchase several years of back issues to generate an idea about the treatments recently researched and discussed. Issues from the mid-1990s were more useful, on average, than issues in the late 90's. Since the turn of the century, the ATA has once again offered valuable information for the tinnitus sufferer. They are currently funding research projects that run the gamut from outstanding to mediocre value per dollar spent. Tell them you are joining on the recommendation of this book. In the United States, I do not recommend any other tinnitus associations.

For Canadians, there is the Tinnitus Association of Canada., which offers a very inexpensive publication. Contact Elizabeth Eayrs at:

Tinnitus Association of Canada
23 Ellis Park Road
Toronto, ON Canada M6S 2V4
phone 416-762-1490
website www.kadis.com/ta/tinnitus.htm
email sandrow@tyenet.com

In the U.K., you can contact the British Tinnitus Association. Membership is 5 pounds. 8 pounds overseas. This includes a quarterly publication called *Quiet.*

British Tinnitus Association
4th Floor, White Building
Fitzalon Square
Sheffield, S1 24Z, UK
phone +44 (0) 11429 6600
toll free phone within UK 0800 018 0527
website www.tinnitus.org.uk

Hearing Loss Organizations & Governmental Agencies

Do you have trouble hearing or know someone who does? Hope For Hearing has been helping the hard of hearing and the deaf for decades. They can be reached at:

Hope For Hearing Foundation
6535 Wilshire Boulevard, Suite 255
Los Angeles, CA 90048
phone 323-651-2615
fax 323-651-2631
web site http://hope4hearing.org
email director@hope4hearing.org

Hearing loss has altered many careers in the music industry. H.E.A.R. can help you save your hearing. A non-profit founded by musicians and physicians and other music professionals, H.E.A.R. offers information about hearing loss, testing, and hearing protection. They will send you an information packet for a small fee.

H.E.A.R. (Hearing Education & Awareness for Rockers)
Box 460847
San Francisco, Ca. 94146
phone 415-409-EARS (3277)
fax 415-409-LOUD (5683)

web site *www.hearnet.com*
email *hear@hearnet.com*

Other organizations that may be useful include:

National Institute of Deafness and Other Communication Disorders
National Institutes of Health
31 Center Drive, MSC 320
Bethesda, MD 20892-2320
phone 301-496-7243
TTY 301-402-0252
website www.nidcd.nih.gov

Vestibular Disorders Association
(support and information for people with head injuries & inner ear disturbances)
Box 4467
Portland, Or. 97208-4467
503-229-7705
503- 229-8064 (fax)
website www.vestibular.org
email veda@vestibular.org

Hyperacusis Network

Hyperacusis, also known as phonophobia, tends to respond more quickly to therapeutic interventions than does tinnitus. If you find yourself afraid or offended by certain sounds regardless of volume, you experience hyperacusis. Almost always, hyperacusis can be reduced with hypnotherapy and/or various medications. You may contact me for further information about reducing severe hyperacusis. An excellent newsletter with past issues available is published by Don

Malcore, a kind soul who has dedicated much of the past several years to helping those with hyperacusis.

> *Hyperacusis Network*
> *Attention: Don Malcore*
> *444 Edgewood Dr.*
> *Green Bay, Wisconsin 54302-4873*
> *website www.hyperacusis.net*
> *email hyacusis@netnet.net*

Mr. Malcore publishes a useful quarterly publication and has a loyal audience of readers. Tell Don this book recommended that you become a member. He can provide most or all of the back issues he has published for a very nominal fee.

Day by Day – Your Healing Process

Each day for the first 21 days of your healing process, then one day each week and, later, one day each month, I urge you to make a log of the volume of your tinnitus, the distress you felt that day (or week or month), and other components of your lifestyle that may be affecting your tinnitus. Please keep excellent records for yourself and for your health practitioner. You make your physician's job much simpler if you are prepared when you see her or him. Remember, your doctor cannot hear your tinnitus.

By keeping an easy to read chart, such as the one that follows for you to keep daily, weekly and monthly, you will provide important information to your health professionals and have greater personal insights into your healing process. After the first few weeks pass there is no reason to keep a daily record of your tinnitus. After the first few months there is no longer a need to keep a weekly record of your tinnitus. After six months, there is no need to keep records any longer. This exercise is part of the habituation. You are paying attention to the noise purposefully at first, then gradually allowing it to be less important.

Do not assume that, just because two weeks pass, all of your days will be quieter and calmer than they were two weeks ago. You will, in all likelihood, progressively get better with fewer bad days per week, as time goes on.

At least five times each day in the first three weeks, record the time of the reading. Then record how loud your tinnitus is on a scale of one–to–five or one–to–ten. Then record how distressed or depressed you are, using the same system. Next describe what foods, herbs, and medications you are using in the space provided. This will help you discover if there is anything you are consuming that is exacerbating your tinnitus. Once you have collected one week's worth of information, you can begin recording data onto a weekly chart and graphing your improvement. Eventually you will set aside this entire journal and find that it is no longer necessary to track your tinnitus, as all likelihood, it will have quieted dramatically or you will have become habituated to it if it persists. That will be a day to celebrate, and I will celebrate with you, as I do with every client who heals and finds the way to an improved quality of life.

TIME OF DAY	VOLUME LEVEL	DISTRESS LEVEL	MEDICATIONS, HERBS, REMEDIES, FOODS CONSUMED
Nighttime			
Wakeup			
Morning			
Noon			
Afternoon			
Dinner			
Evening			
Bedtime			
Comments about today			

The Last Word

Ninety–nine out of every one hundred people who read this book, then go out and pursue every effective avenue discussed in this book will be equipped to either reduce the volume of their tinnitus, reduce the emotional distress associated to tinnitus, or both. The odds that you will enjoy a far better quality of life two years from now are overwhelmingly in your favor.

Every therapy has a drawback. It may be side effects, inconvenience, or financial investment. I spent over $10,000 and 2-$^1/_2$ years of my life getting better... and it was worth every penny! Peace of mind is worth the persistence, patience, and investment it took. If you need help, call my office and I will attempt to help you in any way possible. Godspeed.

Key Points to Remember in This Chapter

- Stress, Panic Disorder, Anxiety, Depression and/or Emotional Problems (SPADE) can predispose individuals to suffer when tinnitus onsets
- Reducing SPADE often means reducing tinnitus volume and normally means reducing the suffering component from tinnitus.
- 78 percent of people with tinnitus have suffered a virtual lifelong prevalence of depression in contrast to 21 percent of control groups in one recent study. (Control groups attempt to represent a more general population for comparison in studies like this.)
- 60 percent of people with tinnitus are currently suffering from depression compared to 7 percent in control groups in a recent study.
- Individuals with depression and tinnitus suffer from three times as many other physical ailments as do those in control groups.
- Personality traits attributed to tinnitus sufferers in significantly greater proportion than the "normal" population include introspectiveness, rumination, feeling like a victim, and tendencies to hostile response.
- Always rule out the possibility of a tumor by getting an MRI or CT scan before beginning therapy or treatment for tinnitus.
- Tinnitus Habituation Therapy (Auditory Habituation) is effective long-term therapy in reducing the distress of tinnitus in over 80 percent of individuals.

- Anti-anxiety medications are effective in about 70 percent of tinnitus sufferers in reducing volume and distress.
- Hypnotherapy is effective in reducing volume and distress in about 70 percent of sufferers. However, this success level is practitioner dependent, meaning the practitioner needs to be experienced in working with tinnitus patients for success levels to be met.
- One herb, Ginkgo Biloba, helps about one third of individuals with central tinnitus reduce volume.
- Never try to ignore your tinnitus. Always try to focus on other stimuli.
- Joining a Tinnitus Association is a good way for you to know that you are not alone with tinnitus.
- Keeping a Day by Day Report of your progress helps you see that over the long term you are emotionally feeling better and realize the volume of your tinnitus is lowering.

CHAPTER SIX
Tinnitus: Looking Back and Looking Forward

I remember the day I woke up and the tinnitus was gone. It was Christmas time in 1995. After 30 months of living in hell, one morning I experienced silence. The maddening noise had completely vanished, and did not recur until August of 1996. Since then, it has returned a few times per month, for a couple of hours at a time—usually at bedtime, after a long and stressful day.

By 1996, my life took a profound turn away from selling, into a life of seeing clients with tinnitus and helping them in my role of psychotherapist–hypnotherapist. I had not intended to go in this direction, but when I "went silent," so many people suffering with tinnitus wanted the answer. In response to thousands of phone calls, emails, faxes, and letters, I began writing articles and posting information about tinnitus relief on my website at http://www.kevinhogan.com/.

The purpose of this chapter is to share my conclusions about tinnitus therapy and treatment, based on my experience with hundreds of clients, thousands of consultations, and continuous leviathan correspondence over the past six years. I cannot answer every question about tinnitus, nor offer a new scientific theory. I can tell you what I know is helping people turn the volume down. I will also speculate about future research and where more answers may be

Where does tinnitus originate?

Many questions are still unanswered as to *where* tinnitus exists in the human body. The initial thought many people have is that it is somewhere in the ear. There is no doubt in my mind that in some people, this is true. Perhaps otoacoustic emissions from the ear send noisy signals to the brain and that is tinnitus. Perhaps. In some cases this is very possible.

There is one thing about which we can be certain. In all cases, tinnitus is experienced in the brain and interpreted by the brain. In other words, like physical pain, tinnitus is interpreted and, to some extent, generated in the brain. After years of doing psychotherapy and hypnotherapy with people who suffer from tinnitus, my experience is that it can, and often does go away with the right program, the right treatment plan.

Imagine that there are hundreds of highways in your brain. (There are billions, but if you can imagine a map of your country with all of the interstate highways visible, that's enough to understand this useful metaphor.) These highways, when interconnected, form memory and allow you to think and create. There are probably no other thought centers in the body. There are probably no other creative thinking centers in the body. The neural circuitry, the *highways,* are where it's all at.

> In all cases, tinnitus is experienced in the brain and interpreted by the brain

Think of someone you love. Think about your loved one in great detail: what your loved one looks like, sounds like, maybe even how your loved one feels. Just do this for a moment before continuing. Your "conscious self" just took an off ramp from reading this article to an image or sound or feeling, or all three, connected to someone you love. The "driver of your car," *you,* went from reading this chapter to someone you love. This act literally lit up an entirely different set of circuits and neural pathways in your brain.

- Some of these highways have tinnitus "on them."
- Some of these highways do not have tinnitus "on them."

These two statements are certain. They are not hypotheses, nor are they theories. These statements are facts.

It is interesting to note that there is some evidence that some cases of tinnitus are caused by an instability of the structure of the cells in some parts of the brain.

My years of experience using different kinds of hypnosis with hundreds and hundreds of clients, along with case studies from colleagues such as Ron Stubbs, Dianne Olson, and others, offer further insights about the origin of tinnitus.

■ In regression hypnosis, when clients are directed to times in their life when tinnitus was not present, almost all clients do not hear their tinnitus while in trance.[1] This can be for periods of time up to two hours during our session work. During these two hours, most clients do not hear their tinnitus at all. They are driving themselves along highways that do not have tinnitus "on them." This is consistently true. At least 70 percent, and as many as 90 percent of clients report this experience.

■ In regression hypnosis, when clients are regressed to describe incidents of serious events where tinnitus volume is loud and distressing, they almost always experience increased tinnitus and distress. Upon relating these incidents many times in trance, the client's anxiety and helplessness reduce, and often the client experiences little or no anxiety to loud tinnitus while in trance.

■ When clients are brought out of trance and are attentive to everything else in the world, their tinnitus tends to be louder (although this is not always true) for an hour or two, then it remits significantly, often to levels that are substantially quieter than when the client walked into the office.

---

1 TRANCE refers to a focused state of attention in which the client is only attentive to what they are directed to be attentive of. There is nothing mysterious about trance. If you cry at the end of It's A Wonderful Life with Jimmy Stewart and Donna Reed, you are in trance because you have dissociated from the real world and bought into the world of the Baileys and the evil Mr. Potter.

■ Long–term results show significant gains in almost all cases. Now, this is a sticky point. Clients who faithfully do their homework and practice all of the different focusing and self–hypnosis exercises we assign do substantially better than those who fly into town for three days, leave, and do nothing at home. Personal responsibility is critical.

■ Meditation, for people with moderate to severe tinnitus, has proven largely ineffective.

■ Hypnosis that relies on relaxation and calming techniques has almost no value when contrasted with guided imagery. But...

■ Imagery is a distant second place when contrasted with the long–term results of the hypnotic interventions mentioned in the first two bullet points.

The Goal of Tinnitus Therapy

We have yet to see a documented case wherein a client improved dramatically after one session of hypnotherapy of psychotherapy. Generally speaking, 15 hours or more of therapy are necessary. It takes some time to get those big eight–lane highways in the brain to atrophy into dirt roads that are rarely traveled. That, by the way, is the goal of tinnitus therapy. The objective and focus of the therapist should always be to: (a) desensitize the client to the sound of tinnitus; and (b) teach the client how to focus on other experiences in life—past, present, or future—that do not have "tinnitus on the highway."

The good news is that most cases of tinnitus, regardless of cause, improve with time, therapy, and plenty of successfully completed homework. The bad news is that there are not a lot of therapists out there who understand how to work with people suffering from tinnitus.

More Good News: Approaches That Work

- Clients continue to respond favorably to medications such as Zoloft, Effexor, and Paxil (antidepressants).
- Clients also tend to respond as well or better to Xanax and Ativan (anti-anxiety medications).
- Clients have also reported positive results with Neurontin and Klonopin (anti-convulsants).

The number of medications that help tinnitus sufferers reduce volume and suffering is so great that it is a shame that the FDA (to my knowledge) still has not approved medications for tinnitus sufferers.

A medication that reduces the fear response helps extinguish the fear response to tinnitus, and thus, the amount of attention paid to tinnitus (thereby shrinking the 8–lane highway into 6 or 4 or fewer lanes). Long–term use of anti-anxiety medication is probably warranted for most severe cases, The resultant fewer suicides and long-term positive change likely supercede the minor side effects and remote possibilities of addiction to these medications.

Those medications that reduce depression, obsession, and compulsive behaviors will also continue to help those suffering with tinnitus. The SSRIs tend to most effective, in my experience, but other medications certainly can help as well.

The Osteopath

Many people complain that their tinnitus is exacerbated by pressure on their forehead, different head positions, and teeth clenching. When I hear this, I immediately refer the person to an osteopath (D.O., or Doctor of Osteopathy).

For some reason, osteopathic treatment, **Intracranial Sacral Therapy,** seems to be effective in helping a majority of my clients who report these exacerbating elements. I can't explain all of the reasons why, though I do have hypotheses. The human body generally responds well to touch and feelings of connectedness. Perhaps there is some of this mindbody response in the client's experience. Perhaps the human body can become so stressed and distressed that it changes brain chemistry. Perhaps the sphenomandibular ligament that connects the area of the ear drum to the jaw is causing some kind of pressure in the ear, like plucking a guitar string.

One client named John was planning to come to Minnesota to work with me. I sent him to a local D.O. and he never needed to keep his appointment with me. Regular treatments by his osteopath were all he needed for elimination of tinnitus. I've had similar situations with clients in which I did a telephone consultation and suggested other treatments such as Prozac, Zoloft, and Xanax.

Auditory Habituation

Tinnitus Retraining Therapy is a fancy phrase for auditory habituation. I've talked with many people who have improved by using sound generators. I've spoken with many others who couldn't stand to have the little noise makers in their ears.

What I have found nearly universal in acceptance by clients is listening to classical music, environmental sounds, and new age music that both soothes and creates a secondary sound source for attention. Auditory habituation is a *must* for tinnitus remission and recovery.

I strongly suggest that all of my clients play music in the background all do long or, at least, keep a television on. Anything that provides about 50 decibels of sound will do the trick. People with severe hyperacusis will need to start at 40 decibels and work their way up, over time, to 50 decibels.

These Usually Don't Help

As time has gone by I have seen fewer cases of people improving from any kind of tinnitus sound with ginkgo. For a while I thought gingko might be a significant part of the therapeutic regime for most clients. Today, I suggest that clients talk to their medical doctors about ginkgo, but I can't recommend it evangelically, as I did five years ago.

I've also seen very few cases of people improving with homeopathic remedies and acupuncture. None of the bogus drops and mail order "medications" showed any improvement that I could find.

Changes in diet have rarely seemed to help tinnitus sufferers, in my experience, nor have herbal potions and remedies.

The Future

In the long term, "they" almost certainly will not find a single cure for tinnitus because tinnitus has so many etiologies (causes). Tinnitus is experienced in so many ways that it seems like aggressive multimodal treatment programs will continue to be in the best interest of the average tinnitus sufferer. What these clients will find is that tinnitus can be greatly reduced in most cases through desensitization and alternative attention therapies.

The Multi–Modal Approach That Works

For years I have advocated a multi-modal approach to tinnitus therapy, and that has proven to be right on the mark. For the average client suffering with severe tinnitus, I recommend the following, in order of importance:

1. Talk to your doctor immediately about starting a fairly long–term treatment plan with low doses of anti-anxiety medications such as Xanax, Klonopin, or Ativan.
2. Talk with the same doctor about starting a fairly long–term treatment plan with moderate daily use of SSRI medications.
3. Listen to music or the television all day as background noise. Avoid silence and extremely loud places. If you can't do this, see an audiologist and buy a pair of sound generators that are comfortable for you to wear.
4. Begin hypnotherapy with someone who has a great deal of experience with tinnitus.
5. Begin psychotherapy with someone who has a great deal of experience with tinnitus.

6. Begin using self–hypnosis tapes for alternative attention and focusing practice. Use the tapes every day. (We can help you with this: See our catalog at the website: http://www.kevinhogan.com/)

7. See an osteopath for 5 sessions. After 5 sessions, you are likely to know if this is one of the keys for you. (Hint: Those clients with the best success are those whose tinnitus is much louder when they are lying down on the floor or in bed.)

8. Avoid support groups and other people who want to talk about their tinnitus all day long. Once you have an action plan, unless you are a therapist or doctor, avoid others who want to focus on their tinnitus. Tinnitus, in some respects, is an "attention disorder."

9. Start living a life that is rich and filled with the things you love to do today! If that tinnitus were a wake–up call to happiness, today would be the day to answer the call.

Evolution of Tinnitus Research:
A Limited Chronological Bibliography
& Abstracts

1994-Present

1. Mattox, Douglas E, and Jastreboff, Pawel.
    "Tinnitus Habituation Therapy: The University of Maryland Tinnitus and
    Hyperacusis Center Experience." *International Tinnitus Journal*, 3.1 (1997): 31–
    32.

2. Shulman, Abraham.
    "A Final Common Pathway for Tinnitus- The Medial Temporal Lobe System."
    International Tinnitus Journal, 1.2 (1995): 115-126.

3. Ehrenberger, K.; Denk, D.; and Felix, D.
    "Receptor Pharmacological Models for Causal Tinnitus Therapy."
    Otorhinolaryngologia Nova (1995): 148–152

4. Ehrenberger, K., and Felix, D.
    "Receptor Pharmacological Models for Inner Ear Therapies with Emphasis on
    Glutamate Receptors: A Survey." *Acta Otolaryngol* (Stockh) 115, (1995): 236–
    240.

5. Podoshin, L.Y.; Ben–David, Fradis M.; Malastkey, S.; and Hafner H.
    "Idiopathic Subjective Tinnitus Treated By Amitriptyline
    Hydrochloride/Biofeedback." *International Tinnitus Journal* 1.1 (1995): 54-60.

6. Werner, J.F.; Richter B.; Laubert, A.
    "Some Remarks on the Classification of Subjective Idiopathic Tinnitus (SIT) –
    An Essay Toward Establishing a Cross-Matched Grading System." *International
    Tinnitus Journal* 1.1 (1995): 39–41.

7. Sweetow, Robert W.
    "Evolution of Cognitive-Behavioral Therapy as an Approach to Tinnitus Patient
    Management." *International Tinnitus Journal* 1.1 (1995): 61–65.

8. Henry, Jane L, and Wilson, Peter H.
    "Coping with Tinnitus: Two Studies of Psychological and Audiological
    Characteristics of Patients with High and Low Tinnitus-Related Disorders."
    International Tinnitus Journal, 1.2 (1995).

9. Werner, J.F.; Richter, B.; and Laubert, A.
    "Some Remarks on the Classification of Subjective Idiopathic Tinnitus – An
    Essay Toward Establishing a Cross-Matched Grading System." *International
    Tinnitus Journal*, (1995): 1.1: pp. 38–40.

10. Kraft, Joseph.
    "Hyperinsulinemia: The Common Denominator of Subjective Idiopathic Tinnitus
    and other Idiopathic Central and Peripheral Neurootological Disorders."
    International Tinnitus Journal 1.1 (1995): pp. 46–53.

11. Shulman, A., and Strashun A.
    SPECT Imaging of the Brain and Tinnitus. Presented at the Fourth International
    Seminar Inner Ear Medicine and Surgery, (Jul 1994) Snowmass, CO.

12. Lipton, S.A., and Rosenberg PA.
    "Excitatory Amino Acids as a final common pathway for neurological disorders.
    Mechanisms of Disease." *New England Journal of Medicine*, 330.9: (9 Mar
    1994): 613–622.

13. Shulman A.
    "Stress Model for Tinnitus." in *Proceedings of XXI Scientific Meeting of the NES.*
    Vol XXII. (1994) Bad Kissingen, Germany.

14. Shulman A., and Strashun A.
    "SPECT Imaging of Brain and Tinnitus." case reports in *Cerebral SPECT
    Imaging*. Edited by V. Heertum and A. Tikofsky. Raven Press (1994): 210–212.

15. Frick G.S.; Strashun A.; Aronson F.; Kappes R.; and Shulman A.
    "The Scintigraphic Appearance at Pathophysiological Loci in Central Type
    Tinnitus: An Tc99m - HMAPO Study." Abstract JNM (Suppl), (May 1993): 210.

16. Jastreboff Pawell J., and Hazell J.W.P.
    "A neurophysiological approach to tinnitus: clinical implications." Br J Audio l
    27 (1993): 7–17.

Historical: 1993 and Older

1. Gilbert, Gordon J.
    "Pentoxifylline–induced musical hallucinations." *Neurology* 43.8 (Aug
    1993):1621–1622.

ABSTRACT: Describes the case of a severely deaf 88 yr old woman who presented
after having experienced 2 wks of almost constant musical auditory
hallucinations. A few days before the onset of the hallucinations, her otologist
had prescribed pentoxifylline for tinnitus. The hallucinations stopped when the
pentoxifylline was discontinued.

2. Alster, Jason. Shemesh, Zecharia. Ornan, Michael. and Attias, Joseph.
    "Sleep disturbance associated with chronic tinnitus." *Biological Psychiatry* 34
    (Jul 1993): 84–90.

    ABSTRACT: Assessed the reported prevalence and severity of sleep disturbance in
    80 chronic tinnitus patients without major psychiatric disturbances. Subjects'
    tinnitus was associated with noise–induced permanent hearing loss. Mini Sleep
    Questionnaire (MSQ) sleep disturbance scores of 77 percent of the patients were
    higher than those of 30 male normal controls. Highest MSQ scores in patients
    with a sleep complaint were for delayed sleep, morning awakenings, mid–sleep
    awakenings, morning fatigue, and chronic fatigue. Self–rated severity of the
    tinnitus was greater in patients with higher sleep disturbance scores. Also, self–
    rated depressive symptomatology was highly correlated with sleep disturbance.
    Retrospective examination of sleep records and polysomnographic data for 10
    patients with a complaint of chronic tinnitus revealed a combined effect for the
    tinnitus condition when associated with another conventional sleep disorder.

3. Brennan, James F.; Byrnes, John J.; Jastreboff, Pawel J.
    "Salicylate–induced phantom auditory effects on reinforced behavior in pre- and
    postweanling rats." *Psychobiology* 21:1 (Mar 1993): 60–68.

    ABSTRACT: Two experiments explored normal hearing or salicylate– (SAL)
    induced phantom auditory perception in young rats. 24 hrs prior to training in
    Exp 1, 45 male preweanling pups (14-21 days of age) were exposed to continuous
    background noise. They were injected with sodium SAL or saline before or after
    training to suppress approach responses to a lactating dam during noise offset
    periods. The sequence of injection initiation affected acquisition and extinction
    rates, and the oldest Subjects behaved similarly to adults reported in studies of
    SAL–induced auditory effects (P. J. Jastreboff et al, 1988). Adapting the task in
    Exp 2 for 18 male postweanling pups 32 days of age produced greater
    suppression and prolonged extinction when SAL was administered prior to
    acquisition and extinction sessions, whereas Subjects injected with saline before
    training and SAL before extinction showed rapid recovery from suppression.

4. Gordon, A. G.
    "Benzodiazepines and the ear: Tinnitus, hallucinations and schizophrenia."
    Canadian Journal of Psychiatry 38.2 (Mar 1993): 156–157.

    ABSTRACT: Discusses implications of M. Fisman's (see PA, Vol 79:12794) case
    of benzodiazepine–precipitated musical hallucinations. The case clarifies how
    drugs act nonspecifically on the ear, suggests a nonspecific physiological action
    of trigger auditory hallucinations, and sheds light on the pathogenesis of
    schizophrenia.

5. Goebel, G., and Hiller, W.
    "Psychische Beschwerden bei chronischem Tinnitus: Erprobung und Evaluation
    des Tinnitus-Fragebogens (TF). [Psychological complaints in chronic tinnitus:
    characteristics and evaluation of the Tinnitus.]" *Verhaltenstherapie* 2.1 (Mar
    1992): 13–22. Language: German.

    ABSTRACT: Studied psychological complaints in patients with chronic tinnitus to
    assess the psychometric properties of a German version of the TQ by R. S.

Hallam et al (1988). Subjects were 138 adults (aged 20–74 yrs) with chronic tinnitus. Subjects' responses to the 52 TQ items were analyzed to determine the frequency of specific psychological complaints. The instrument's factorial structure, dimensions, subscale intercorrelations, internal consistency, and criterion validity were also analyzed. (English abstract)

6. Attias, Joseph; Shemesh, Zecharya; Sohmer, Haim; Gold, Shlomit; et al. Comparison between self–hypnosis, masking and attentiveness for alleviation of chronic tinnitus. *Audiology* 32.3 (May–Jun 1993): 205–212.

ABSTRACT: The efficacy of self–hypnosis (SH), masking (MA), and attentiveness (AT) to the patient's complaints in the alleviation of tinnitus was evaluated. 45 male patients (aged 34–53 yrs) with chronic tinnitus related to acoustic trauma were assigned to 3 matched subgroups: SH, AT, or MA. The therapeutic stimuli in the SH and MA sessions, recorded on audio–cassettes, were given to the patients for use when needed. SH significantly reduced the tinnitus severity; AT partially relieved the tinnitus; MA did not have any significant effect. (French abstract)

7. Katon, Wayne; Sullivan, Mark; Russo, Joan; Dobie, Robert; et al. "Depressive symptoms and measures of disability: A prospective study." *Journal of Affective Disorders* 27.4 (Apr 1993): 245–254.

ABSTRACT: Hypothesized that decreases in severity of depressive symptoms in patients with chronic tinnitus would correlate with reductions in measures of functional disability (FD). The correlations were described between several measures of FD and Hamilton Rating Scale for Depression scores in 38 patients with major depression and 54 patients with depressive symptoms. Most measures of FD decreased synchronously with Hamilton Depression Scale scores in both groups of Subjects. Subjects whose depression improved had a significantly greater change in each disability measure. Results suggest that there was a significant correlation between improvement in both major depression and depressive symptoms, and decreases in measures of FD in an aging population with a chronic medical illness.

8. Hallberg, Lillemor R.; Johnsson, Tommy; and Axelsson, Alf. "Structure of perceived handicap in middle-aged males with noise–induced hearing loss, with and without tinnitus." *Audiology* 32.2 (Mar–Apr 1993): 137–152.

ABSTRACT: By using a modified stepwise regression analysis technique, the structure of self–perceived handicap and tinnitus annoyance in 89 males with noise–induced hearing loss was described. Handicap was related to 3 clusters of variables reflecting individual, environmental, and socioeconomic aspects. 60 percent of the variance in self–perceived handicap was explained by the representatives of these clusters: "acceptance of hearing problems," "social support related to tinnitus," and "years of education." Tinnitus had no impact of its own on self–perceived handicap, and only a modest portion (36 percent) of the variance in tinnitus annoyance was explained by "sleep disturbance" and "auditory perceptual difficulties." (French abstract)

9. Hazell, Jonathan W.; Jastreboff, Pawel J.; Meerton, Leah E.; Conway, Mike J.
    "Electrical tinnitus suppression: Frequency dependence of effects." *Audiology*
    32.1 (Jan–Feb 1993): 68–77.

ABSTRACT: Evaluated electrical stimulation through a round window electrode in
9 patients with unilateral deafness and severe tinnitus. Three Subjects were
permanently implanted, with positive long–lasting results. Analysis of the
threshold of sound perception, tinnitus suppression, and auditory discomfort
levels as a function of current frequency revealed the advantage of low frequency
stimulation. In 2 patients, the loudness of electrically evoked sound perception
was balanced against tones in the hearing ear. Results can be interpreted as
indicating that processes other than auditory masking are responsible for
electrical tinnitus suppression. (French abstract)

10. Landry, Pierre, and Latour, Judith.
    "Neuroleptic malignant syndrome in communicating hydrocephaly and
    microcephaly." *Journal of Clinical Psychopharmacology* 13.1 (Feb 1993): 72–74.

ABSTRACT: Describes the case of a 74–yr–old woman with nausea, dizziness, and
tinnitus who was treated with haloperidol (HAL) when she became increasingly
restless and disoriented. HAL was discontinued for fear of neuroleptic malignant
syndrome when she showed extrapyramidal symptoms. Microcephaly, marked
bilateral ventricular enlargement secondary to cerebral atrophy, and signs of
communicating hydrocephaly were seen on the computerized tomography (CT)
scan. Autopsy showed neuronal changes compatible with Alzheimer's disease
(AD).

11. Risey, John; Briner, Wayne.
    "Dyscalculia in patients with vertigo." *Journal of Vestibular Research:
    Equilibrium & Orientation* 1.1 (1990–91): 31–37.

ABSTRACT: Reports that 14 patients presenting with a primary complaint of
vertigo skipped and displaced decades when asked to count backwards by two.
The error occurred at each decade except the transition from 12 to 8. Compared
with a control group of 7 patients complaining of vertigo, and a 2nd control group
of 8 patients with a primary complaint of tinnitus, the dyscalculia group also
performed the worst at visually recognizing errors, and had the lowest scores on
the arithmetic and digit span portions of the Wechsler Adult Intelligence Scale
(WAIS). Results are discussed with reference to the vestibular/auditory system
and higher cognitive function.

12. McKee, G. J., and Stephens, S. D.
    "An investigation of normally hearing subjects with tinnitus." *Audiology* 31.6
    (Nov–Dec 1992): 313–317

ABSTRACT: In a replication of G. Barnea et al (1990), the hearing sensitivity and
psychological profile of 18 adults with tinnitus and normal hearing was
investigated. Pure–tone and high–frequency audiometry, notched–noise tests,
auditory–brainstem responses, evoked otoacoustic emissions, and the Crown–
Crisp Experiential Index were used to investigate evidence of cochlear
dysfunction in ears with normal hearing thresholds to support a theory of a
peripheral origin of tinnitus. In agreement with Barnea et al, psychoacoustical and

brainstem tests were comparable to those of 19 normally hearing adults without tinnitus. Otoacoustic emissions were worse in ears of tinnitus Subjects, suggesting that tinnitus Subjects had minor cochlear damage. Neurotic personality traits were stronger in the tinnitus Subjects. (French abstract)

13. Kemp, Simon, and George, Richard N.
     "Masking of tinnitus induced by sound." *Journal of Speech & Hearing Research* 31.5 (Oct 1992): 1169–1179.

     ABSTRACT: In 2 experiments, 8 listeners (aged 21–38 yrs) used external sound to mask the tinnitus induced by a 95–db SPL tone presented for 1 min. Wider bandwidth noises were more effective maskers than were noises of critical bandwidth, which, in turn, were more effective than tonal maskers. Contralateral maskers were often effective, but less so than ipsilateral maskers. Tuning curves showed some degree of frequency specificity that was not related to the frequency of the tinnitus–inducing tone. There were consistent and pronounced differences between individual listeners. Results indicate both similarities and differences between the masking of induced tinnitus and the masking of pathological tinnitus.

14. Hallberg, Lillemor R.; Erlandsson, Soly I.; Carlsson, Sven G.
     "Coping strategies used by middle-aged males with noise-induced hearing loss, with and without tinnitus." *Psychology & Health* 7.4 (Oct 1992): 273–288.

     ABSTRACT: Examined general coping strategies and specific communication strategies, used by 72 adult males with noise-induced hearing loss. 26 Subjects had mild tinnitus, 24 had severe tinnitus, and 22 were without tinnitus. Subjects with severe tinnitus differed in general coping from Subjects without. Subjects with severe tinnitus reported significantly more "escape coping" and "active coping" than did Subjects without tinnitus. The use of specific communication strategies did not differ significantly between groups.

15. Koshes, Ronald J.
     "Use of amitriptyline in a patient with tinnitus." *Psychosomatics* 33.3 (Summer 1992): 341–343.

     ABSTRACT: Presents the case of a 69–yr–old woman who presented with symptoms of depression 6 mo after the onset and diagnosis of tinnitus. After initiating treatment with amitriptyline, the Subject's tolerance for the ringing in her ears seemed to increase, as did her sleep and appetite.

16. Penner, M. J.; Bilger, R. C.
     "Consistent within–session measures of tinnitus." *Journal of Speech & Hearing Research* 35.3 (Jun 1992): 694–700.

     ABSTRACT: Used 2 psychophysical methods, a method of adjustment (MOA) and a forced-choice double-staircase adaptive procedure (FCDS), to measure the predominant pitch and loudness of tinnitus for 11 Subjects during 1 test session. The FCDS within–session variability (WSV) of matches to tinnitus pitch was smaller than for the MOA and comparable to the WSV obtained when the FCDS procedure was used to match objective stimuli that approximated the frequency and level of the tinnitus. The WSV of matches to tinnitus loudness was nearly identical for the FCDS and the MOA and comparable to the WSV obtained when the FCDS procedure was used to match objective stimuli that approximated the frequency and level of the tinnitus. For 3 male Subjects who participated in 20 sessions, the 2 methods produced correlated measures of tinnitus that tracked each other between sessions. This suggests that tinnitus may be stable within a brief time span but fluctuant in the long run.

17. Erlandsson, Soly I.; Hallberg, Lillemor R.; Axelsson, Alf.
     "Psychological and audiological correlates of perceived tinnitus severity."
     Audiology 31.3 (May–Jun 1992): 168–179.

ABSTRACT: Investigated the relationship between tinnitus severity and perceived attitudes, social support, and disability/handicap in a clinical population of 163 Subjects (aged 21–89). Audiological descriptives comprised pure–tone average, etiology of hearing loss, duration of tinnitus, and tinnitus localization. Perceived severity of tinnitus was assessed with a questionnaire focusing on tinnitus impact on aspects of quality of life, concentration, and sleep. Severity was related to perceived attitudes. The influence of social support on severity did not seem to be crucial. More women than men experienced vertigo and unilateral localization. Subjects with multiple localizations were older and had more sleep disturbance than Subjects with tinnitus localized to the ears only. The frequency of headaches was correlated with the severity of tinnitus. (French abstract)

18. Hiller, Wolfgang, and Goebel, Gerhard.
     "A psychometric study of complaints in chronic tinnitus." *Journal of Psychosomatic Research* 36.4 (May 1992): 337–348.

ABSTRACT: Studied the dimensions of psychological complaints due to chronic and disabling tinnitus by means of the Tinnitus Questionnaire (appended) of R. S. Hallam et al (see PA, vol 76:9073) administered to 138 tinnitus sufferers (aged 20–74 yrs) admitted to a psychosomatic hospital. Tinnitus–related patterns of emotional and cognitive distress, intrusiveness, auditory perceptual difficulties, sleep disturbances, and somatic complaints can be differentiated. Scales are proposed for the questionnaire that can be used in clinical and scientific work to specifically assess major areas of tinnitus–related distress and their degree of severity.

19. Jakes, S. C.; Hallam, R. S.; McKenna, L.; Hinchcliffe, R.
     "Group cognitive therapy for medical patients: An application to tinnitus."
     Cognitive Therapy & Research 16.1 (Feb 1992): 67–82.

ABSTRACT: Patients distressed by tinnitus (perceptions of noise[s] in the head/ears) were randomly allocated to 1 of 5 treatments: aural masker, placebo masker, waiting list, group cognitive therapy (GCT), or GCT plus masker. At follow–up (3 mo and 1–2 yrs), only Subjects receiving GCT (with or without a masker) were significantly improved over baseline on a tinnitus distress questionnaire. Irrational beliefs about tinnitus were modified in the baseline period only in Subjects receiving an explanatory booklet about cognitive therapy. These beliefs continued to change from baseline to follow–up only in GCT. Measures of general affective state changed little and not to a significantly greater extent in GCT than in other conditions. Overall results indicate a specific effect of GCT on tinnitus distress not observed in alternative treatments.

20. Halama, Peter.
"Erfahrungen mit der Hypnose-Therapie bei ambulanten Patienten, die unter Tinnitus leiden. Vergleichende Pilotstudie. [Hypnotherapy in patients who are suffering from buzzing in the ear (tinnitus): A comparing]." *Experimentelle und Klinische Hypnose* 8.1 (1992): 49–69. Language: German.

ABSTRACT: Studied the effectiveness of hypnotherapy in the treatment of drug–resistant tinnitus. Subjects were 80 adults with tinnitus. The 50 Subjects in the hypnotherapy group were treated with a combination of individual hypnosis, group hypnosis, and self–hypnosis. The 30 Subjects in the control group received either the standard pharmacotherapy or no treatment. Changes in the intensity of tinnitus were assessed during the 1st 3 mo of hypnotherapy and at 12–mo and 24– mo follow–ups. Intergroup differences were analyzed. (English abstract)

21. Nilsson, Sune; Axelsson, Alf; and De, Gu Li.
"Acupuncture for tinnitus management." *Scandinavian Audiology* 21.4 (1992): 245-251.

ABSTRACT: Investigated 3 parameters of tinnitus (intensity, annoyance, and awareness) in 56 Subjects with tinnitus who were treated with acupuncture. Three patients reported improvement lasting for 10 days posttreatment; 6 Subjects described their tinnitus as worse. Estimated improvement rate (consistent for all 3 parameters) was 20 percent, while the corresponding deterioration rate was 25 percent. Statistical analysis of the whole group showed no general treatment effects. Additional side effects were reported by 33 percent of the Subjects. More Subjects reported positive (24 percent) than negative (16 percent) effects. These effects were mainly of a psychological or psychosocial nature, attributed to group processes and the intervention itself. Decreased anxiety was mentioned by 28 percent of the Subjects.

22. Bauer, Peter; Korpert, Karl; Neuberger, Manfred; Raber, Alfred; et al.
"Risk factors for hearing loss at different frequencies in a population of 47,388 noise–exposed workers." *Journal of the Acoustical Society of America* 90.6 (Dec 1991): 3086–3098.

ABSTRACT: Examined hearing thresholds in 47,388 noise–exposed workers to determine the relationship between risk for hearing loss and different variables across a number of tonal frequencies. Data were gathered from audiometric screening tests conducted by the Austrian Workers' Compensation Board. Multilinear regression analysis showed that the influences of age, sex, noise dosage, hearing protector usage, head injuries, ear diseases, and tinnitus act additively on predicting pure-tone hearing threshold and that a 4,000-Hz threshold may be used as an early indicator of noise-induced hearing damage. Only the intercorrelational coefficient between age and noise dosage was significant.

23. Settle, Edmund C.
"Tinnitus related to bupropion treatment." *Journal of Clinical Psychiatry* 52.8

(Aug 1991): 352.

ABSTRACT: Describes cases of tinnitus related to bupropion treatment in a 50–yr–old woman and a 52–yr–old woman. In both cases, the tinnitus ceased when the drug was withdrawn.

24. Hughes, John R.; Higgins, Stephen T.; Bickel, Warren K.; Hunt, William K.; et al. "Caffeine self-administration, withdrawal, and adverse effects among coffee drinkers." *Archives of General Psychiatry* 48.7 (Jul 1991): 611–617.

ABSTRACT: Examined caffeine self-administration, withdrawal, and adverse effects among 22 coffee drinkers (aged 19–61 yrs). Reliable caffeine self–administration occurred in 3 of 10 coffee drinkers in Study 1 and 7 of 12 coffee drinkers in Study 2. Headaches, drowsiness, and fatigue were reported more frequently on decaffeinated (3 mg caffeine) coffee days than on caffeinated (100 mg caffeine) coffee days during the withdrawal and adverse effects period. Occurrence of headaches on substitution of decaffeinated coffee prospectively predicted subsequent caffeine self-administration. Subjects who consumed 400–500 mg of caffeine during the withdrawal and adverse effects period reliably reported stomachache, sweating, talkativeness, tinnitus, and tremulousness.

25. Cochrane, Gordon J.
    "Client-therapist collaboration in the preparation of hypnosis interventions: Case illustrations." *American Journal of Clinical Hypnosis* 33.4 (Apr 1991): 254–262.

ABSTRACT: Presents case studies of 4 patients (aged 23–73 yrs) to illustrate client–therapist collaboration in the development of effective heterohypnosis in a surgical setting and audiotape–assisted self–hypnosis for performance anxiety, tinnitus, and situational depression. In each case, the clients demonstrated sufficient capacity for absorption and sufficient ego–strength to respect and use his/her own contributions.

26. Goebel, Gerhard; Keeser, Wolfgang; Fichter, Manfred; Rief, Winfried.
     "Neue Aspekte des komplexen chronischen Tinnitus-Teil I: Uberprufung eines multimodalen verhaltensmedizinischen Behandlungskonzeptes. [New aspects of complex chronic tinnitus: I. Testing a multimodal.]" *Psychotherapie Psychosomatik Medizinische Psychologie* 41.3–4 (Mar–Apr 1991): 115–122. Language: German.

ABSTRACT: Used a multidimensional psychophysiologic tinnitus model integrated with multimodal behavior therapy. Human subjects: 28 male and female German adults (aged 29–72 yrs) (chronic tinnitus). Tests used: The Hopkins Symptom Checklist, Freiburg Personality Inventory, and Tinnitus Questionnaire (R. R. Coles and R. S. Hallam, 1987). Treatments: cognitive therapy, operant therapy, emotional therapy, physical therapy, family therapy, sociotherapy, and physical perception. (English abstract)

27. Goebel, Gerhard; Keeser, Wolfgang; Fichter, Manfred; Rief, Winfried.
    "Neue Aspekte des komplexen chronischen Tinnitus-Teil II: Die verlorene Stille: Auswirkungen und psychotherapeutische Moglichkeiten beim komplexen chronischen Tinnitus. [New aspects of complex chronic tinnitus: II]."
    Psychotherapie Psychosomatik Medizinische Psychologie 41.3–4 (Mar–Apr

1991): 123–133. Language: German.

ABSTRACT: Discusses the following topics: epidemiology and pathophysiology of tinnitus; psychotherapy of complex chronic tinnitus; and parallels between tinnitus and the chronic pain syndrome. Psychological variables in chronic tinnitus and the use of cognitive, behavioral, emotional, and interactional therapy components are considered. (English abstract)

28. Wilson, Peter H.; Henry, Jane; Bowen, Maitland; Haralambous, George.
     "Tinnitus Reaction Questionnaire: Psychometric properties of a measure
     of distress associated with tinnitus." *Journal of Speech & Hearing Research* 34.1
     (Feb 1991): 197–201.

ABSTRACT: Describes the development, reliability, factor analysis, and validity of
the Tinnitus Reaction Questionnaire (TRQ), a scale designed to assess the
psychological distress associated with tinnitus. Psychometric analyses of the TRQ
were examined with a total of 156 Subjects (aged 24–80 yrs) in 3 samples.
Results indicate very good test–retest reliability and internal consistency. Factor
analysis yielded 4 factors that were interpreted as General Distress, Interference,
Severity, and Avoidance. Moderate to high correlations were found between the
TRQ and clinician ratings and self–report measures of anxiety and depression,
but a low correlation was found with neuroticism. The TRQ provides a useful
index of distress related to tinnitus for selection of Subjects and clinical
assessment and may be useful as a measure of change in coping ability.

29. Halford, Jonathan B., and Anderson, Stewart D.
     "Anxiety and depression in tinnitus sufferers." *Journal of Psychosomatic
     Research* 35.4–5 (1991): 383–390.

ABSTRACT: 112 members (aged 29–87 yrs) of a tinnitus self-help group
completed psychological assessments of anxiety and depressive tendency and a
tinnitus severity questionnaire. Tinnitus was associated with elevated anxiety trait
and depression, although the coefficients were of low magnitude. Advancing age
(65+ yrs) was related to a reduction in depressive tendency; being male was
associated with lower anxiety and depression scores.

30. Carlsson, Sven G., and Erlandsson, Soly I.
     "Habituation and tinnitus: An experimental study." *Journal of Psychosomatic
     Research* 35.4–5 (1991): 509–514.

ABSTRACT: Examined whether variation in suffering among individuals with
about the same amount of tinnitus would be due to differences in habituation to
the perceived sound. 14 patients (mean age 61 yrs), including 7 complainers and
7 noncomplainers, participated in an experiment in which changes in skin
conductance and heart–rate responses to a series of tinnitus-like sound stimuli
were studied. No group differences in habituation were observed, although
complainers scored higher on measures of anxiety and amount of fears. This
finding suggests that complainers are more psychologically vulnerable than
noncomplainers. Facilitatory processes (e.g., disinhibition) may be more
important than deficient habituation for the inability in some individuals to adapt
to their tinnitus.

31. Sevigny-Skyer, Solange C.; Dagel, Delbert D.
"Deafness simulation: A model for enhancing awareness and sensitivity among hearing educators." *American Annals of the Deaf* 135.4 (Oct 1990): 312–315.

ABSTRACT: Describes a deafness simulation project implemented by a college for deaf students to help hearing faculty and staff members improve their awareness of deafness and their sensitivity toward deaf students. Participants are fitted with tinnitus maskers that produce a constant sound similar to a running shower, resulting in a 72–decibel loss in both ears. 48 participants rated the experience on a scale of 1 (most negative) to 10 (most positive). The average rating was 9.5.

32. Berthaux, Paul.
"Le traitement des premiers signes de declin cerebral: etude de l'efficacite et de l'acceptabilite de Duxil chez 12,548 patients. [Medication of the early stages of cerebral deterioration: A study]. *Psychologie Medicale* 22.9 (Sep 1990): 935–945. Language: French.

ABSTRACT: Studied the efficacy and acceptability of Duxil with 12,548 50–75 yr old outpatients, whose clinical files were collected from all French regions. Subjects were treated for memory and attention impairments or sensory neuropathic disorders, combined with one or more cerebrovascular risk factors. Memory and concentration improved in 70 percent of Subjects after 2–mo treatment; improvements in headaches, vertigo, and tinnitus were equally significant. Clinical and biological acceptability of the drug is excellent; side effects are rare and consist mostly of digestive disorders. Results of this multicenter study confirm the dual–therapy benefits brought by Duxil in enriching the blood with oxygen, relieving symptoms immediately, and protecting patients from cerebrovascular risks because of its oxygen–diffusing capacity at the cerebral and neurosensory level. (English abstract)

33. Stouffer, James L., and Tyler, Richard S.
"Characterization of tinnitus by tinnitus patients". *Journal of Speech & Hearing Disorders* 55.3 (Aug 1990): 439–453.

ABSTRACT: Surveyed 235 female and 293 male tinnitus patients (aged 14–88 yrs) to obtain their reactions to tinnitus. Tinnitus was present for more than 26 days per month in 74 percent of the Subjects. Hearing levels at 1,000 and 4,000 Hz were <=25 dB HL for 18 percent of the Subjects, suggesting that some had normal hearing or mild hearing losses. Prevalence of tinnitus in Subjects with noise–induced hearing loss was 30 percent for males; 3 percent for females. About 25 percent of the Subjects reported tinnitus severity had increased since tinnitus onset. Effects were more severe in Subjects who reported tinnitus as their primary complaint and in Subjects having Meniere's syndrome tinnitus. Some Subjects reported that noise exacerbated their tinnitus, others that a quiet background exacerbated it.

34. Jastreboff, Pawel J.
"Phantom auditory perception (tinnitus): Mechanisms of generation and perception." *Neuroscience Research* 8.4 (Aug 1990): 221–254. Pub type: Literature Review: Review.

ABSTRACT: Analyzes the phenomenon of tinnitus (TN) from the point of view of general neurophysiology. Existing theories and their extrapolation are presented, together with new mechanisms of TN generation. These mechanisms involve Ca and Ca channels in cochlear function and have implications for malfunction and aging of the auditory and vestibular systems. TN may result from the perception of activity that cannot be induced by any combination of external sounds. Signal recognition and classification circuits, working on holographic or neuronal network-like representation, may be involved in the perception of TN and may be subject to plastic modification. All levels of the nervous system may be involved in TN.

35. Kirsch, Cynthia A.
"A controlled group outcome study on the effects of self-regulatory treatments of tinnitus." Dissertation, *Dissertation Abstracts International* 50.12–B, Pt 1 (Jun 1990): 5884.

36. Katon, Wayne; Sullivan Mark D.
"Depression and chronic medical illness." *Journal of Clinical Psychiatry* 51.6 (Jun 1990 Supp): 3–11. Pub type: Literature Review: Review.

ABSTRACT: Reviews placebo–controlled, double-blind treatment studies to illustrate that major depression (MDP) accompanying chronic medical illness (CMI), chronic pain, and comorbidity is amenable to treatment with antidepressants. Epidemiology studies show that 15–33 percent of medical inpatients suffer from affective disorder compared to 2–4 percent of the general population. A community study showed that patients with one or more CMIs had a 41 percent increase in the relative risk of having any recent psychiatric disorder. Other studies found a high prevalence of MDP in patients with cancer, neurologic illnesses, cardiac disease, and rheumatoid arthritis. Also highlighted are studies on health care utilization, functional disability, and somatization; risks of lack of diagnosis and treatment; increased mortality; and treatment of patients with MDP and medical illness. Chronic tinnitus is suggested as a model for research into comorbidity in MDP and medical illness.

37. Collet, L.; Moussu, M. F.; Disant, F.; Ahami, T.; et al.
"Minnesota Multiphasic Personality Inventory in tinnitus disorders." *Audiology* 29.2 (Mar–Apr 1990): 101–106.

ABSTRACT: Examined the relation between Minnesota Multiphasic Personality Inventory (MMPI) and tinnitus in 100 Subjects (aged 19–82 yrs) with tinnitus disorders. The overall profile of tinnitus sufferers on the MMPI was normal. Higher scores on the depression scale were obtained in males. High hypochondria scores were related to long duration of tinnitus. High psychoasthenia scores were associated with hearing loss. Despite an analogy previously described between chronic pain and tinnitus, the psychometric parameters of tinnitus and of headaches are quite different. (French abstract)

38. Hollander, Eric; DeCaria, Concetta M.; Schneier, Franklin R.; Schneier, Holly A.; et al.
"Fenfluramine augmentation of serotonin reuptake blockade antiobsessional treatment." *Journal of Clinical Psychiatry* 51.3 (Mar 1990): 119–123.

ABSTRACT: Administered open treatment with fenfluramine augmentation (FA) to 7 patients (aged 28–53 yrs) with obsessive–compulsive disorders. These Subjects had only a partial response to, or experienced side effects with, 5–hydroxytryptamine (5–HT) or serotonin reuptake blockers (fluoxetine, fluvoxamine, or clomipramine). In doses of 20–60 mg/day, FA was well tolerated and resulted in a further decrease in obsessions and compulsions in 6 Subjects. Possible side effects of FA are increased sexual arousal, impotency, or tinnitus.

39. Pearson, Heather J.
"Interaction of fluoxetine with carbamazepine." *Journal of Clinical Psychiatry* 51.3 (Mar 1990): 126.

ABSTRACT: A 55–yr–old woman with major depression (MD) and grand mal seizures and a 45–yr–old woman with MD and multiple sclerosis, taking stable doses of the tricyclic anticonvulsant carbamazepine (CZ), demonstrated both increased plasma concentrations of CZ (fluorometric assay) and associated adverse side effects (e.g., diplopia, blurred vision, tremor, vertigo, nausea, vomiting, tinnitus) following the administration of fluoxetine.

40. Feder, Robert.
"Tinnitus associated with amitriptyline." *Journal of Clinical Psychiatry* 51.2 (Feb 1990): 85–86.

ABSTRACT: Reports on a 23–yr–old male who developed tinnitus (TN) during 3 wks of treatment for depression with amitriptyline (AMI). A week after AMI was discontinued, the Subject's TN was gone. The Subject refused further antidepressant treatment, but made satisfactory progress with psychotherapy alone. The case suggests that AMI should be added to the list of tricyclic antidepressants that can cause TN.

41. Attias, Joseph; Shemesh, Zecharya; Shoham, Chaya; Shahar, Amnon; et al.
"Efficacy of self-hypnosis for tinnitus relief." *Scandinavian Audiology* 19.4 (1990): 245–249.

ABSTRACT: Randomly assigned 36 males (aged 28–58 yrs) with tinnitus (TT) to 1 of 3 treatment conditions: self hypnosis (SH), presentation of a brief auditory stimulus (BAS) to the ear with TT, or no–treatment waiting list control. 73 percent of SH Subjects reported disappearance of TT during treatment sessions, as compared with only 24 percent of BAS Subjects. Following treatment, the short–term (1 wk) and long–term (2–mo) symptom profiles of only SH Subjects revealed a significant improvement. SH may be a beneficial method for the relief of TT.

42. George, Richard N., and Kemp, Simon.
"Investigation of tinnitus induced by sound and its relationship to ongoing tinnitus." *Journal of Speech & Hearing Research* 32.2 (Jun 1989): 366–372.

ABSTRACT: Tinnitus was temporarily induced by monaurally presented sound, and its level monitored using a dichotic loudness–matching task. Exp 1 with 6 normal–hearing Subjects found no effect of varying the level, bandwidth, or center frequency of an inducing noise on the level or duration of the induced tinnitus. Exp 2 investigated tinnitus induced by a 1–kHz, 95–dB SPL tone in 53 Subjects (aged 18–35 yrs) with thresholds in the normal range but with varying degrees of ongoing tinnitus that ranged from no discernible sound sensation at all, through an apparently normal but usually inaudible noise or ringing, to constant or near–constant tinnitus. Results suggest that some kinds of ongoing tinnitus may arise from the auditory process responsible for induced tinnitus.

43. Farber, Shereen D.
"Living with Meniere disease: An occupational therapist's perspective." Special Issue: Motor control. *American Journal of Occupational Therapy* 43.5 (May 1989): 341–343.

ABSTRACT: Reports the case of a female occupational therapist who developed Meniere disease, a condition whose sequelae may consist of vertigo, tinnitus, episodic hearing loss, or visual symptoms. The therapist's professional background enabled her to learn self–taught, new movement patterns (involving excessive fixation and decreased segmentation) that enabled her to accomplish necessary daily living tasks. A battery of vestibular and audiometric tests produced no definitive findings. After a conservative 6–wk treatment of salt restriction, the therapist was greatly improved.

44. Reich, Gloria E.
"Direct and indirect costs of tinnitus: Factors for decisionmaking." Dissertation. *Dissertation Abstracts International* 49.10–B (Apr 1989): 4257.

45. Laird, Lyle K.; Lydiard, R. Bruce.
"Imipramine–related tinnitus." *Journal of Clinical Psychiatry* 50.4 (Apr 1989): 146.

ABSTRACT: Presents the case of a 38–yr–old woman with a history of depression who developed tinnitus while receiving imipramine (IMI) in a 6–wk, double-blind, placebo-controlled trial of fluvoxamine vs IMI. The tinnitus resolved without adjustment of the IMI dose or discontinuance of the drug and did not recur.

46. Kirsch, Cynthia A.; Blanchard, Edward B.; Parnes, Steven M.
"Psychological characteristics of individuals high and low in their ability to cope with tinnitus." *Psychosomatic Medicine* 51.2 (Mar–Apr 1989): 209–217.

ABSTRACT: 77 adults (aged 19–75 yrs) with tinnitus were assessed with a variety of standardized psychological tests and scales assessing subjective loudness, annoyance, and ability to cope with the tinnitus. Significant correlations were found between coping ability and psychological test scores. Based on their responses on the coping scale, Subjects were classified as high or low copers. The 2 tinnitus groups were also compared to a group of 34 chronic pain (headache) patients (aged 16–68 yrs) and to a group of 65 nonheadache/nontinnitus controls (aged 21–64 yrs). Results revealed that the low coping tinnitus Subjects were significantly more psychologically distressed than the high copers. Low copers were similar in their psychological profiles to the chronic pain patients, while high copers were similar to the nonpatient controls.

47. Kirsch, Cynthia A.; Blanchard, Edward B.; Parnes, Steven M.
"A review of the efficacy of behavioral techniques in the treatment of subjective

tinnitus." *Annals of Behavioral Medicine* 11.2 (1989): 58–65. Pub type: Literature Review: Review.

ABSTRACT: Presents a critique of several of the major studies that have assessed the efficacy of relaxation and/or biofeedbacktreatments in the treatment of subjective tinnitus. The methodological problems of many of the studies reviewed limit confidence in their results with regard to treatment effectiveness. It is suggested that some of the positive results obtained in these studies may have been due to the use of global measures of posttreatment success. The goal of research in this area should be to develop effective treatments that take into account cognitive and psychological factors, as well as patient characteristics that may affect treatment outcome.

48. Lindberg, Per; Scott, Berit; Melin, Lennart; Lyttkens, Leif.
    "The psychological treatment of tinnitus: An experimental evaluation."
    Behaviour Research & Therapy 27.6 (1989): 593–603.

ABSTRACT: Treated disabling tinnitus in 27 patients (aged 19–82 yrs) in an experimental setting with 2 different types of therapy aiming at the development of coping behavior. One was focused on behavioral control procedures, while the other aimed at more cognitive control methods such as distraction. Assessments of subjective loudness, discomfort from tinnitus, and controllability were made on analog scales before treatment and at a questionnaire follow–up. Psychoacoustic measures such as personal loudness units were used with these self–recordings and for evaluation of treatment effects. Results confirm favorable reports on behavioral methods in tinnitus. However, no differences were found between therapies. Findings are discussed in light of coping and adaptation theory (R. S. Lazarus and S. Folkman, 1984).

49. Erlandsson, Soly; Carlsson, Sven G.; Svensson, Anders.
    "Biofeedback in the treatment of tinnitus: A broadened approach." *Goteborg Psychological Reports* 19.6 (1989): 12.

ABSTRACT: Describes the use of biofeedback (BFB) training in a 56–yr–old man with severe tinnitus of 2 yrs duration. Forehead area electromyogram (EMG) BFB training substantially reduced symptom intensity. The relationship between the therapeutic effect and the cognitive and emotional changes observed are discussed. The author argues that the model of BFB training should include a broad array of therapeutic mechanisms. In the treatment of tinnitus and other placebo–sensitive disorders, nonspecific BFB treatment factors may exemplify higher levels of G. Schwartz's (1984) hierarchical arrangement of mechanisms contributing to BFB–aided therapeutic changes. These include (1) education and insight and (2) motivation and attitude change.

50. Tyler, Richard S.; Stouffer, James L.; Schum, Robert.
    "Audiological rehabilitation of the tinnitus client." *Journal of the Academy of Rehabilitative Audiology* 22 (1989): 30–42.

ABSTRACT: Describes a plan for the treatment of tinnitus (TNS) that includes (a) initial counseling, (b) handicap evaluation, (c) psychoacoustical measurement, and (d) in–depth counseling. The initial counseling session involves determining the severity of the client's TNS and providing information about TNS. The handicapping nature of TNS can be determined in more detail with an open-ended problems questionnaire or a TNS handicap scale. In some situations it is useful to measure TNS pitch, loudness, and its masking and postmasking characteristics. Audiologists can fit hearing aids and TNS maskers to reduce TNS and can provide cognitive behavior-modification therapy.

51   Jastreboff, Pawel J.; Brennan, James F.; Coleman, John K.; Sasaki, Clarence T. "Phantom auditory sensation in rats: An animal model for tinnitus." *Behavioral Neuroscience* 102.6 (Dec 1988): 811–822.

ABSTRACT: To measure tinnitus induced by sodium salicylate injections, 84 rats were used in a conditioned suppression paradigm. In Exp 1, Subjects were trained with a conditioned stimulus/stimuli (CS) consisting of the offset of a continuous background noise. One group began salicylate injections before Pavlovian training, a 2nd group started injections after training, and a control group received daily saline injections. Resistance to extinction was profound when injections started before training but minimal when initiated after training, suggesting that salicylate–induced effects acquired differential conditioned value. In Exp 2, salicylate treatments were mimicked by substituting a 7 kHz tone in place of respective injections, resulting in effects equivalent to salicylate–induced behavior. A 3rd experiment included a 3 kHz CS, and again replicated the salicylate findings. In Exp 4, motivational level was decreased, and the sequential relation between salicylate–induced effects and suppression training was retained. Findings support the demonstration of phantom auditory sensations in animals.

52.   Penner, M. J.
"Judgments and measurements of the loudness of tinnitus before and after masking." *Journal of Speech & Hearing Research* 31.4 (Dec 1988): 582–587.

ABSTRACT: Explored the relation between changes reported in the perception of the loudness of tinnitus after noise exposure and changes measured in matches to the loudness of tinnitus after noise exposure in 6 persons with hearing loss. Pre-exposure assessment of the loudness of tinnitus was followed by monaural exposure to broadband Gaussian noise (for a 5–min period), after which a pulsed, 200–msec tone was presented either ipsilateral or contralateral to the exposed ear. Following each noise exposure, Subjects (a) judged the change in the pre- and postexposure tinnitus strength and (b) compared the loudness of the postexposure tinnitus to that of the pure tone. For 3 Subjects, pre- and postexposure magnitudes did not differ significantly even though the judgments indicated that the pre- and postexposure loudness of the tinnitus had changed. Data suggest that some loudness judgments may reflect variability in the perceived strength of tinnitus rather than the effect of noise on tinnitus.

53.   Busto, Usoa; Fornazzari, Luis; Naranjo, Claudio A.
"Protracted tinnitus after discontinuation of long-term therapeutic use of benzodiazepines." *Journal of Clinical Psychopharmacology* 8.5 (Oct 1988): 359–362.

ABSTRACT: Reports 3 cases of protracted tinnitus associated with benzodiazepine (BZD) withdrawal in male patients (aged 57, 34, and 49 yrs) without tinnitus prior to the time they began to use BZDs. In one Subject, a single case, double–blind, randomized experiment was performed that compared the effect of diazepam and placebo on the occurrence and severity of tinnitus.

54. Hallam, R. S.; Jakes, S. C.; Hinchcliffe, R.
"Cognitive variables in tinnitus annoyance." *British Journal of Clinical Psychology* 27.3 (Sep 1988):213-222.

ABSTRACT: 79 clinic outpatient adults who reported tinnitus completed 2 questionnaires devised to investigate dimensions of complaint. Following a factor analysis of data provided by the 1st questionnaire, the 2nd questionnaire included questions concerning coping attitudes and beliefs about tinnitus. Results indicate the presence of 3 main dimensions of complaint: emotional distress, auditory perceptual difficulties, and sleep disturbance. Several smaller factors suggest that complaint was more complex than originally predicted. The 2nd questionnaire successfully discriminated complaining from noncomplaining Subjects.

55. Reich, James H.; Noyes, Russell; Yates, William.
"Anxiety symptoms distinguishing social phobia from panic and generalized anxiety disorders." *Journal of Nervous & Mental Disease* 176.8 (Aug 1988):510-513.

ABSTRACT: Compared 14 social phobic, 18 generalized anxiety disorder, and 48 panic disorder patients on 4 categories of anxiety symptoms (autonomic hyperactivity, muscular tension, vigilance, and apprehensive expectation). Six specific symptoms (palpitations, chest pains, tinnitus, blurred vision, headaches, fear of dying, and dry mouth) distinguished social phobia from panic disorder, while 4 (headaches, fear of dying, sweating, and dyspnea) distinguished social phobia from generalized anxiety disorder. Most symptom differences were in the autonomic hyperactivity category of symptoms. Findings further confirm the validity of social phobia as a distinct disorder.

56. Sullivan, Mark D.; Katon, Wayne; Dobie, Robert; Sakai, Connie; et al.
"Disabling tinnitus: association with affective disorder." *General Hospital Psychiatry* 10.4 (Jul 1988):285-291.

ABSTRACT: 40 adults with disabling tinnitus (DT) and 14 controls (CTLs) complaining of hearing loss completed a structured psychiatric interview, the SCL–90, a chronic illness problem inventory, and a revised ways of coping checklist. Findings reveal that DT Subjects had a significantly greater lifetime prevalence of major depression and a significantly higher prevalence of current major depression than CTLs. Currently depressed DT Subjects had significantly higher scores on all subscales of the SCL–90 compared with the nondepressed DT Subjects and CTLs. Results demonstrate that DT was strongly associated with major depression.

57. Penner, M. J.
"The effect of continuous monaural noise on loudness matches to tinnitus." Journal of Speech & Hearing Research 31.1 (Mar 1988):98-102.

ABSTRACT: Data from 2 psychophysical tasks are presented. In the 1st task, 8 Subjects with sensorineural hearing loss and tinnitus adjusted the intensity of a continuous monaural noise to mask the tinnitus; in the 2nd in the presence of continuous monaural noise, the same Subjects adjusted the intensity of a pulsed monaural tone to match the loudness of the tinnitus. The tone was either ipsilateral or contralateral to the noise. Although the noise level required to mask the tinnitus increased substantially, as did the level of the ipsilateral matching tone, the change in the level of the contralateral matching tone was minimal. The functioning of the peripheral auditory system is discussed.

58. Jakes, S.
"Otological symptoms and emotion: A review of the literature. Advances in Behaviour Research & Therapy 10.2 (1988):53–103. Pub type: Literature Review; Review.

ABSTRACT: Reviews the literature on emotional aspects of otological symptoms (primarily hearing loss, vertigo, and tinnitus), which are common and often disabling. It is estimated that 35 percent of the population reports a hearing disorder. Two issues are addressed: (1) Is emotional disturbance associated with hearing loss, tinnitus, or vertigo and (2) If so, is that distress the cause or effect of those symptoms?

59. Lindberg, Per.
"Effects of self–control training on tinnitus in a deaf patient: a case study." Scandinavian Journal of Behaviour Therapy 17.3–4 (1988):223–229.

ABSTRACT: Describes the treatment of a 26–yr–old deaf woman with severe tinnitus, using a behavioral approach that included relaxation and various forms of behavioral and cognitive coping strategies. The patient received therapy in 5 1–hr sessions during which specially adapted methods like the use of sign interpretation, visual prompts, and written instructions were used. Positive results in various self–reports made both after treatment and at a 5–mo follow–up are discussed.

60. Spencer, Marlene; Mulcahy, Robert.
"Biofeedback as a technique for the study of tinnitus: a case study." *Canadian Journal of Rehabilitation* 1.2 (1987 Winter):111–118.

ABSTRACT: Examined whether either of the 2 basic characteristics of subjective tinnitus (loudness and pitch) could be altered. Temperature training using visual biofeedbackwas given to a 62–yr–old male post–acoustic neuroma S. Despite establishment of good digital temperature control, earlobe temperature control was not established. However, session warming of the earlobe did occur, indicating that regular increase in blood circulation to the area could be induced without medication. (French abstract)

61. Kirsch, Cynthia A.; Blanchard, Edward B.; Parnes, Steven M.
"A multiple–baseline evaluation of the treatment of subjective tinnitus with relaxation training and biofeedback." *Biofeedback & Self Regulation* 12.4 (Dec 1987): 295-312.

ABSTRACT: Six adults with subjective tinnitusreceived training in relaxation techniques and electromyogram (EMG) and thermal biofeedbackin a multiple-baseline across–Subjects design. Daily tinnitus disturbance and sleep disturbance diaries were kept throughout. Audiological and psychological evaluations were made at various treatment phases. At posttreatment assessment, Subjects also completed global ratings of their perceived improvement in ability to cope with the tinnitus, stress caused by the tinnitus, and severity of the tinnitus, as well as their overall satisfaction with the treatment. Ratings on the global scales were generally very positive. By way of contrast, the daily diary results revealed little if any treatment effect.

62. Leader, Leslie.
"Psychological aspects of tinnitus: the effects of attentional focus, anxiety, and fatigue." DISSERTATION. Dissertation Abstracts International 48.1–B (Jul 1987): 267.

63.   Danenberg, Mary A.; Loos-Cosgrove, Margaret; LoVerde, Marie.
"Temporary hearing loss and rock music." *Language, Speech, & Hearing Services in Schools* 18.3 (Jul 1987 Jul):267–274.

ABSTRACT: Pre- and postexposure binaural pure–tone air–conduction thresholds were obtained for 2,000, 4,000, and 6,000 Hz from 20 12–17 yr old students and 7 adults at a live rock–music concert. 19 students and 6 adults experienced at least a 5 db threshold shift at 1 or more frequencies, with significant average threshold shifts at all frequencies. 15 students and all the adults who experienced shifts also reported tinnitus. Of the 6 Subjects selected to be retested 3 days postexposure, 4 demonstrated only partial recovery to preexposure thresholds.

64.   Penner, M. J.
"Maskingof tinnitus and central masking." *Journal of Speech & Hearing Research* 30.2 (Jun 1987):147-152.

ABSTRACT: Considered external stimuli that mask tinnitus and investigated whether the tinnitus is masked centrally (retrocochlearly) or peripherally (in the cochlea), using 3 patients with tinnitus and sensorineural hearing losses and 3 normal–hearing observers. Results show that, for the patients, masking was primarily dependent on intensity. For Subjects with normal hearing, the central masking of a continuous tone was primarily dependent on the intensity of a contralateral masker; masking was nearly independent of masker frequency. Implications of the flat tuning curves on the design of tinnitus maskers and an interpretation of the similarity of tinnitus masking and central masking are discussed.

65.   Tandon, Rajiv; Grunhaus, Leon; Greden, John F.
"Imipramine and tinnitus." *Journal of Clinical Psychiatry* 48.3 (Mar 1987): 109–111.

ABSTRACT: Presents 5 case vignettes of patients (aged 23–55 yrs) who developed tinnitus when treated with imipramine (150–250 mg/day). Subjects were identified in a chart review of 475 patients treated in an affective disorder clinic with tricyclic antidepressants. Tinnitus subsided within 2–4 wks without any specific treatment.

66.   Kearney, Brian G.; Wilson, Peter H.; Haralambous, George.
"Stress appraisal and personality characteristics of headache patients:

comparisons with tinnitus and normal control groups." *Behaviour Change* 4.2 (1987): 25–32.

ABSTRACT: Compared 41 headache patients, 25 tinnitus patients, and 39 normal controls on the Neuroticism scale of the Eysenck Personality Questionnaire (EPQ), Manifest Anxiety Scale (MAS), Beck Depression Inventory, Unpleasant Events Schedule, and measures of emotional control and cognitive appraisal of stressors. Subjects were 17–71 yrs old. Headache sufferers scored in the more pathological direction than the controls on the EPQ, MAS, and the measure of cognitive appraisal of stressors. Tinnitus patients did not differ from normal controls on these measures.

67. Haralambous, George; Wilson, Peter H.; Platt–Hepworth, Sarah; et al.
     "EMG biofeedback in the treatment of tinnitus: an experimental evaluation."
     Behaviour Research & Therapy 25.1 (1987): 49–55.

ABSTRACT: 26 tinnitus patients received either electromyogram (EMG) biofeedback with counterdemand instructions, EMG biofeedback with neutral demand instructions, or no treatment. Assessment was conducted on self-report measures of the distress associated with tinnitus, the loudness, annoyance, and awareness of tinnitus, sleep–onset difficulties, depression, and anxiety. Audiological assessment of tinnitus was also conducted and EMG levels were measured (the latter only in the 2 treatment groups). No significant treatment effects were found on any of the measures. There was a significant decrease in the ratings of tinnitus awareness over the assessment occasions, but the degree of change was equivalent for treated and untreated groups. Results do not support the assertion that EMG biofeedback is an effective treatment for tinnitus

68. Ost, Lars–Goran.
     "Applied relaxation: Description of a coping technique and review of controlled studies." *Behaviour Research & Therapy* 25.5 (1987): 397–409.

ABSTRACT: Describes the rationale and practice of applied relaxation (AR), the purpose of which is to teach the patient a coping skill that will enable him/her to relax rapidly to counteract and eventually abort anxiety reactions altogether. A review of 18 controlled outcome studies shows that AR has been used for different phobias, panic disorder, headache, pain, epilepsy, and tinnitus. Results also show that AR was significantly better than no–treatment or attention-placebo conditions, and as effective as other behavioral methods with which it was compared. At follow-ups after 5–19 mo the effects were maintained or further improvements were obtained.

69. Ince, Laurence P.; Greene, Renee Y.; Alba, Augusta; Zaretsky, Herbert H.
     "A matching–to–sample feedback technique for training self-control of tinnitus.
     Health Psychology 6.2 (1987): 173–182.

ABSTRACT: Treated 30 individuals (aged 24–82 yrs) with subjective tinnitus aurium with a matching–to–sample feedback procedure. Subjects' tinnitus sounds were reproduced audiometrically on all characteristics and were presented to them in the noninvolved ear or in both ears when the tinnitus was binaural. This experimental sound was then reduced in 5–db steps within sessions, and Subjects had the task of concentrating on reducing the loudness of their tinnitus until a match was achieved between it and the experimental sound at each new db level. Results show a significant difference in db levels from baseline to final training session. Nearly all Subjects demonstrated a marked reduction in tinnitus loudness, with several eliminating it completely.

70. Harrop-Griffiths, Jane; Katon, Wayne; Dobie, Robert; Sakai, Connie; et al. "Chronic tinnitus: association with psychiatric diagnoses. *Journal of Psychosomatic Research* 31.5 (1987):613–621.

ABSTRACT: 21 consecutive patients with severe tinnitus (TN) were interviewed using the National Institute of Mental Health Diagnostic Interview Schedule and were asked to complete the SCL–90 and the chronic illness problem inventory developed by L. D. Kames et al (see PA, Vol 72:5632). Compared with 14 patients with hearing loss, the TN Subjects had a significantly greater lifetime prevalence of major depression and a significantly higher prevalence of current major depression. The currently depressed TN Subjects had significantly higher scores on all subscales of the SCL–90, except the Phobia and Paranoid subscales, as compared with the nondepressed TN group and on all scales compared with controls. The number of psychosocial problems was significantly greater in the TN group compared with controls and in the currently depressed TN Subjects compared with nondepressed TN Subjects.

71. Lindberg, Per; Scott, Berit; Melin, Lennart; Lyttkens, Leif. "Long-term effects of psychological treatment of tinnitus." Scandinavian Audiology 16.3 (1987):167–172.

ABSTRACT: Reassessed 20 adult patients with severe tinnitus who had undergone behavioral treatment, including applied relaxation and perceptual restructuring 9 mo after treatment. Among the self-recorded variables (tinnitus loudness, discomfort from tinnitus, depression, and irritation), discomfort from tinnitus was the only variable that was still significantly reduced. As part of the 9-mo follow-up assessment, Subjects' recall of the loudness and discomfort from their tinnitus was studied. Correlations between original recordings and recall data were low. Results show that psychological treatment of tinnitus has positive long-term effects.

72. Wilkinson, J. B. "Hypnosis in medicine." BOOK CHAPTER in: *Hypnotherapy: A handbook.* Psychotherapy handbooks series. Michael Heap, Windy Dryden, Eds. Milton Keynes, England: Open University Press (1991): 128–144.

ABSTRACT: (Summarized) Discusses the use of hypnosis in the treatment of a variety of physical disorders and conditions. (from the chapter) hypnotherapeutic approaches: general principles; choice of cases... specific applications: procedures and research findings; the respiratory system (asthma, chronic hyperventilation); the cardiovascular system (angina, palpitation, post-coronary thrombosis rehabilitation, hypertension); the nervous system (migraine, tinnitus); skin conditions (warts, eczema); gastrointestinal conditions (peptic ulcer (gastric and duodenal), irritable bowel syndrome); terminal illness.

73. Bradley, Walter G., ed.; Daroff, Robert B., ed.; Fenichel, Gerald M., ed.; Marsden, C. David, ed. *Neurology in clinical practice, Vol. 1: Principles of diagnosis and management.* Butterworth Heinemann Publishers; Boston, MA, US, (1991). Pub type: Instructional Material; Textbook.

ABSTRACT: (from the preface) We have long felt the need for a practical textbook of neurology that covers all of the clinical neurosciences for neurologists in training and in practice, and for physicians in related disciplines. Such a textbook should provide not only a description of neurological disease and its pathophysiology, but also the practical approach to diagnosis and management that only years of experience can offer.... To be practical, the textbook must assume that the reader already has an understanding of the normal structure and function of the nervous system, and of general medicine. With these goals in mind, and with the help of our many colleagues throughout the world, we have compiled this textbook of neurology. (from the book) The chapters in this section (Section I) cover major symptoms or manifestations that bring a patient to a neurologist.... The chapters in this section (Section II) cover those disciplines that may be termed neurodiagnostic, namely central and peripheral neurophysiology, neuropsychology, and neuroimaging.... The chapters in this section (Section III) provide a brief outline of the clinical neuroscience disciplines that relate to neurology.... The chapters in this section (Section IV) describe the general principles of neurological management; provide a brief outline of the major modalities of treatment, namely pharmacotherapeutics, surgery, and rehabilitation; and discuss the specific management of neurological problems in newborns, pregnant women, and the elderly.
CONTENTS: (Abbreviated).
PART I. APPROACH TO COMMON NEUROLOGICAL PROBLEMS.
Approach to the diagnosis of neurological disease. Walter G. Bradley, Robert B. Daroff, Gerald M. Fenichel and C. David Marsden. (Chapter record available).
Episodic impairment of consciousness. Joseph Bruni. (Chapter record available).
Falls and drop attacks. Bernd F. Remler and Robert B. Daroff. (Chapter record available).
Acute confusional states. Mario F. Mendez. (Chapter record available).
Clinical approach to stupor and coma. Jonathan O. Harris and Joseph R. Berger. (Chapter record available).
Excessive daytime drowsiness. J. David Parkes. (Chapter record available).
Assessing impairments of intellect and memory. Daniel Tranel. (Chapter record available).
Behavior and personality disturbances. Michael R. Trimble. (Chapter record available).
Language disorders. Howard S. Kirshner. (Chapter record available).
The apraxias. Howard S. Kirshner. (Chapter record available).
Disorders of recognition. Antonio R. Damasio and Daniel Tranel. (Chapter record available).
Dysarthria, dysfluency, and dysphagia. David B. Rosenfield and Alberto O. Barroso. (Chapter record available).
Visual loss. Robert L. Tomsak. (Chapter record available).
Abnormalities of the optic nerve and retina. Roy W. Beck. (Chapter record available).
Eye movement disorders and diplopia. Patrick J. Lavin. (Chapter record

available).
Pupillary and eyelid abnormalities. Terry A. Cox. (Chapter record available).
Dizziness and vertigo. B. Todd Troost. (Chapter record available).
Hearing loss and tinnitus without dizziness and/or vertigo. B. Todd Troost, Kenya S. Taylor and Hugh O. Barber. (Chapter record available).
Disturbances of taste and smell. Pasquale F. Finelli and Robert G. Mair. (Chapter record available).
Lower cranial neuropathies. Maurice R. Hanson and Patrick J. Sweeney. (Chapter record available).
Cranial and facial pain. Jerry W. Swanson. (Chapter record available).
Monoplegia. David Goldblatt. (Chapter record available).
Hemiplegic syndromes. Monroe Cole. (Chapter record available).
Paraplegia and quadriplegia. P. D. Thompson. (Chapter record available).
Motor unit weakness. Michael H. Brooke. (Chapter record available).
The hypotonic infant. Gerald M. Fenichel. (Chapter record available).
Sensory abnormalities of the limbs and trunk. Thomas R. Gordon and Stephen G. Waxman. (Chapter record available).
Movement disorder symptomatology. Anthony E. Lang. (Chapter record available).
Ataxic disorders. Anita E. Harding. (Chapter record available).
Brainstem syndromes. Michael Wall. (Chapter record available).
Muscle pains and cramps. Robert B. Layzer. (Chapter record available).
Walking disorders. P. D. Thompson and C. David Marsden. (Chapter record available).
Sexual and sphincter dysfunction. David N. Rushton. (Chapter record available).
Arm and neck pain. Kapil D. Sethi and Thomas R. Swift. (Chapter record available).
Low back and lower limb pain. Walter G. Bradley. (Chapter record available).
PART II. NEUROLOGICAL INVESTIGATIONS.
The place of laboratory investigations in diagnosis and management. Walter G. Bradley, Robert B. Daroff, Gerald M. Fenichel and C. David Marsden. (Chapter record available).
Quantitative diagnostic methods and decision analysis. Dennis Plante. (Chapter record available).
Clinical neurophysiology. Timothy A. Pedley and Ronald G. Emerson; Jun Kimura and Q. Stokes Dickins. (Chapter record available).
Neuropsychology. L. D. Kartsounis and Elizabeth K. Warrington. (Chapter record available).
Neuroimaging. Samuel M. Wolpert. (Chapter record available).
PART III. THE RELATED CLINICAL NEUROSCIENCES.
Neuroepidemiology. John F. Kurtzke. (Chapter record available).
Neurogenetics. Margaret W. Thompson. (Chapter record available).
Neuroimmunology. S. Sriram. (Chapter record available).
Neurovirology. Paul M. Hoffman and John O. Fleming. (Chapter record available).
Neuroendocrinology. Paul E. Cooper. (Chapter record available).
Neuro–opthalmology. Patrick J. Lavin and Barbara M. Weissman; Robert L. Tomsak. (Chapter record available).
Neuro–otology. B. Todd Troost. (Chapter record available).
Neurourology. David N. Rushton. (Chapter record available).

PART IV. PRINCIPLES OF NEUROLOGICAL MANAGEMENT. (Chapter record available).

74. Troost, B. Todd; Taylor, Kenya S.; Barber, Hugh O.
"Hearing loss and tinnitus without dizziness and/or vertigo." BOOK CHAPTER in: Neurology in clinical practice, Vol. 1: Principles of diagnosis and management.; Walter G. Bradley, Robert B. Daroff, Gerald M. Fenichel, C. David Marsden, Eds. Butterworth Heinemann Publishers, Boston, MA, US. (1991): 201-208.

ABSTRACT: (from the chapter) types of hearing loss... examination (pure tone audiometry, tympanometry); symptoms and diagnosis of hearing loss (conductive loss, sensorineural loss, sensory versus neural lesions, central auditory disorders)... tinnitus... evaluation and management (masking, biofeedback, counseling).

10. Tarlow, Gerald.
Clinical handbook of behavior therapy: Adult medical disorders. Brookline Books, Inc; Cambridge, MA, US, 1989. BOOK Pub type: Guide.

ABSTRACT: (from the introduction) The major purpose of this book is to help the mental health clinician assess and treat a variety of problems by behavioral and cognitive–behavioral methods. The problems contained in this first volume (see companion volume-Tarlow (1989) "Clinical Handbook of Behavior Therapy: Adult Psychological Disorders) are ones that may initially come to the attention of a physician, or may require a thorough physical evaluation, prior to treatment by a mental health clinician.
Each chapter in the book follows the same format. The section on assessment strategies suggests different strategies that have been employed, as discussed in the literature. Rating scales and some structured interviews are included in addition to behavioral observations. It is not the purpose of this section to teach differential diagnosis or review the diagnostic criteria of the disorders. The assessment techniques are generally ones that can best be used to assess the severity of a disorder or monitor treatment progress after a diagnosis has been confirmed.... The section on treatment strategies covers the successful behavioral treatments that have been reported in the literature.... There is an emphasis on techniques that can be applied by the typical clinician.... This section does not evaluate the research that has been reported but suggests various treatment options that have been found to be successful, if even for two clinical case studies. Many chapters include detailed descriptions on how the techniques were applied in the research articles. It is also not the purpose of this book to teach basic behavior therapy techniques.... The section at the end of each chapter, "For More Information," provides descriptions of key articles, book chapters, or entire books that would be useful if more in–depth knowledge is desired.... Each chapter has its own reference section and a cross reference to any other related chapters in this volume.
CONTENTS:
Introduction.
Anorexia nervosa.
Anxiety-Stressful medical procedures.
Aphasia.
Asthma.

Blepharospasm.
Bulimia.
Bruxism.
Cancer.
Colitis.
Compliance.
Constipation.
Conversion disorders.
Dental fear.
Diabetes mellitus.
Diarrhea.
Dysmenorrhea.
Fainting.
Genital herpes.
Headache.
Hyperlipidemia.
Hypertension.
Hyperventilation.
Incontinence.
Insomnia.
Irritable bowel syndrome.
Menopausal hot flashes.
Myopia.
Neurodermatitis.
Pain-Acute.
Pain-Chronic.
Raynaud's disease.
Seizure disorders.
Spasmodic torticollis.
Tardive dyskinesias.
Temporamandibular joint dysfunction and pain syndrome.
Tics.
Tinnitus.
Tourette's syndrome.
Type A behavior pattern.
Ulcers.
Urination–Excessive.
Urinary retention.
Vaginismus.
Vomiting.
Writer's cramp.
Appendix A: Case studies.
Excessive daytime sleepiness.
Hives.
Muscle spasm.
Polydipsia.
Psoriasis.
Sleeptalking.
Sleepwalking.
Speaking stomach syndrome.
Vertigo.

76. Greuel, Hans.
Up to the ears: Sudden deafness, vertigo, tinnitus (3rd rev. ed.). NY (US): V.D.G. Publishing Company (1989). BOOK.

ABSTRACT: (from the preface) The author tackles the problems of patients suffering from sudden deafness, vertigo, or tinnitus from a completely new angle. On the one hand he does have a well–founded education as an otorhinolaryngologist; on the other hand he has enjoyed a far broader education, also specialising in psychoanalysis and psychotherapy. His way of seeing, for example, sudden deafness and its therapy is thus not narrowed to that of the ENT (ear, nose and throat)–specialist, but on the contrary, it encompasses the studying of mankind and its problems in coping with modern civilization. The title of this book, a saying whose real meaning is brought back to us, clearly points out the main theme of this book: sudden deafness is not viewed as an illness of the ear — not even as one of the entire auditory organ — but rather as a complication which arises when man, as he has developed during the millions of years of evolution and has adapted himself optimally to his surroundings, is forced into a hypermodern life–style called civilization, a life–style for which he has not been created.... This results in civilization illnesses such as, for example, sudden deafness.

CONTENTS: (Abbreviated).
Preface (by) R. P. Pohl.
Introduction.
Background.
Why "up to the ears."
The inability to regenerate.
On the brink of exhaustion.
Exhaustion.
Conventional treatment.
The psychosomatics of the vestibulocochlear system.
Treatment and prevention.
Case studies.
Bibliography.
Epilogue.

77. Heap, Michael, ed.
Hypnosis: Current clinical, experimental and forensic practices. London: Croom Helm (1988). BOOK EDITED.

ABSTRACT: (from the foreword) This book is an attempt to present a cross–section of serious and informed work in hypnosis in Great Britain and Ireland. Let me stress that this volume is obviously not intended as a comprehensive textbook of hypnosis. Nevertheless, I believe the reader will find the range of topics remarkably broad.. I believe that the volume will be both interesting and instructive to psychologists and behavioural scientists in both the academic and applied fields, medical, dental and psychiatric practitioners, psychotherapists, and other health service professionals. In addition, those working in the legal fields may find sections of the book useful.

CONTENTS:

Foreword.

78. Karle, Hellmut W.A.
     "Hypnosis in the management of tinnitus." BOOK CHAPTER in: *Hypnosis: Current clinical, experimental and forensic practices.* Michael Heap, Ed. London: Croom Helm (1988): 178-185.

     ABSTRACT: (from the chapter) report of clinical trial; effect of going into a hypnotic trance daily appeared to have beneficial effects.

79. Corso, John F.
     "Sensory-perceptual processes and aging." BOOK CHAPTER in: *Annual review of gerontology and geriatrics,* Vol. 7. Annual review of gerontology and geriatrics. K. Warner Schaie, Ed. NY (US): Springer Publishing Co (1987): 29–55.

     ABSTRACT: (from the chapter) various approaches that may be made to offset, in part, sensory–perceptual problems and thereby improve the personal adjustment of the elderly; technological aids; environments; rehabilitation programs... models and theories ...for investigating problems of aging in sensory-perceptual systems... information theory... signal-detection theory... adaptation–level theory... visual system; structural changes in the visual system with age; spatial vison; vigilance; judgments of lines and figures; eye movements; visual masking;

color vision; visual indices of biological aging... audition; structural changes in the auditory system with age; presbycusis; noise exposure and aging effects; tinnitus; speech intelligibility; auditory indices of biological aging.

80. Penner, M. J.
"Tinnitus as a source of internal noise." *Journal of Speech & Hearing Research* 29.3 (Sep 1986): 400–406.

ABSTRACT: For 7 patients with sensorineural hearing loss and tinnitus, pitch and loudness matches were made to the tinnitus. Three normal-hearing Subjects also participated. These matches were followed by measurement of 3 psychometric functions (probability of a correct response as a function of signal level) for pure tones: one in the presumed tinnitus region (i.e., at the average frequency matching the pitch of the tinnitus), one below the minimum frequency of the matches, and one above the maximum frequency of the matches. Results are consistent with the idea that tinnitus is an unstable signal and with the notion that the unstable tinnitus acts as a source of internal noise.

81. Penner, M. J.
"Magnitude estimation and the 'paradoxical' loudness of tinnitus." *Journal of Speech & Hearing Research* 29:3 (Sep 1986): 407–412.

ABSTRACT: Eight patients with continuous tinnitus and sensorineural hearing loss and 2 patients with tinnitus matched external tones to the tinnitus pitch. These matches were followed by (a) magnitude estimates to measure the loudness function of tones at 1 kHz and at the presumed tinnitus frequency (i.e., at the average frequency matching the pitch of the tinnitus); (b) magnitude estimates of the tinnitus itself; and (c) loudness matches of external tones to the tinnitus. The slope of the loudness function at 1 kHz was substantially smaller than the slope at the presumed tinnitus frequency. The magnitude estimates of the tinnitus coupled with intensity matches to the tinnitus provided coordinates that typically were near the loudness function of the external tone used in the intensity match. Because the slope of the loudness function was much greater at the tinnitus frequency than at 1 kHz, the magnitude estimate of tinnitus loudness corresponded to a lower sensation level at that frequency than at 1 kHz. This finding favors the conclusion that rapid changes in loudness of external tones at the tinnitus frequency account for the paradoxical loudness of the tinnitus, a conclusion that is independent of any mathematical description of the loudness function.

82. Jakes, Simon C.; Hallam, Richard S.; Chambers, Christine C.; Hinchcliffe, Ronald.
"Matched and self–reported loudness of tinnitus: Methods and sources of error. *Audiology* 25.2 (Mar–Apr 1986): 92–100.

ABSTRACT: Studied 62 (15–73 yr old) patients who reported tinnitus at the time of their 1st attendance at a neurootology clinic. Loudness matches were obtained both at the frequency of the tinnitus and at 1 kHz. These matches were expressed in db HL, db sensation level, and in units derived from individualized loudness functions measured as personal loudness units (PLUs). Self–reports of the loudness of tinnitus at the time of loudness matching were obtained on 5 scales. Moderate correlations were found between self–reported loudness and some of the scales by which the loudness match was expressed. When the 7 Subjects who had some difficulty with the test procedures were excluded, the correlations between PLU expressions of the matched loudness and certain of the self-report scales were found to be markedly improved. Correlations of traditional expressions of matched loudness with self-report improved to a limited extent. It is concluded that (1) measurement error can appreciably reduce the maximum correlation between the best self-report measure and loudness match measures, (2) PLU conversions of matched loudness data produce the highest correlations with self-report measures of loudness, and (3) explicitly labeled self-report scales produce better correlations with loudness match values than other self-report scales. (French abstract)

83. Kemp, Simon, and Plaisted, Ian D.
     "Tinnitus induced by tones." *Journal of Speech & Hearing Research* 29.1 (Mar 1986):65–70.

ABSTRACT: Monitored the course of noisy–sounding tinnitus induced in 11 normally hearing Subjects following monaural presentation of intense pure tones. The sensation level of a comparison noise, matched in loudness to the tinnitus by the Subjects, was found to increase first rapidly and then slowly before dying away within approximately 90 sec. The peak level of the tinnitus increased with the level of the inducing tone but was unaffected by its duration or frequency; the duration of the tinnitus was positively related to the frequency but not to the level or duration of the tone. Temporary threshold shift measured with pulsed noise generally occurred after, rather than during, the tinnitus. Substantial individual differences, particularly in the duration of the tinnitus, were apparent (e.g., 2 Subjects recorded high levels of tinnitus in the absence of and in response to tonal stimulation).

84. Jakes, S. C.; Hallam, R. S.; Rachman, S.; Hinchcliffe, R.
     "The effects of reassurance, relaxation training and distraction on chronic tinnitus sufferers." *Behaviour Research & Therapy* 24.5 (1986):497–507.

ABSTRACT: Assessed the effects of psychological therapy on tinnitus distress in a 3–factor experiment in which (1) progressive muscle relaxation therapy was compared to progressive muscle relaxation therapy combined with attention–switching training, (2) immediate therapy was compared to delayed therapy, and (3) 2 therapists were compared. Subjects were 12 male and 12 female tinnitus sufferers (mean age 55 yrs). Before treatment, basic information about tinnitus management (including the role of attitudes and beliefs) was provided together with orientation to coping as a goal of treatment. The annoyance caused by tinnitus and the loudness of the tinnitus were rated separately 3 times per day, and insomnia was recorded. The annoyance of tinnitus decreased more rapidly at the beginning of treatment than during the orientation period and continued to decline during therapy. Neither the loudness nor the intrusiveness of the tinnitus declined during therapy. The distress arising from the tinnitus and the activities affected by the tinnitus declined during both orientation and treatment, while effects on insomnia were inconsistent. Results are discussed in relation to a model of tinnitus-annoyance.

85. O'Hanlon, Bill.
"The use of metaphor for treating somatic complaints in psychotherapy." *Family Therapy Collections* 19 (1986): 19–24.

ABSTRACT: Discusses the use of hypnosis and metaphorical techniques in therapy. An indirect approach is often effective for "experience" complaints, those involving affective or somatic difficulties. Case examples are presented of the successful use of metaphors for treatment of somatic problems.

86. Lyttkens, Leif; Lindberg, Per; Scott, Berit; Melin, Lennart.
"Treatment of tinnitus by external electrical stimulation." Scandinavian Audiology 15.3 (1986):157–164.

ABSTRACT: Studied the effect of transcutaneous electrical stimulation on troublesome tinnitus in 5 consecutive patients who were referred to the Audiological Department of the University Hospital in Uppsala, Sweden. Continuous self-recordings of complaints were made throughout the study. Electrical stimulation was found to have a positive effect in 1 Subject, a placebo effect in 1 Subject, and no or a negative effect in 3 Subjects.

87. Allen, James R.
"Salicylate–induced musical perceptions." *New England Journal of Medicine* 313.10 (Sep 1985):642–643.

ABSTRACT: A 70–y–old female suffering from otosclerosis and rheumatoid arthritis with blood level of salicylate (from taking 12 aspirins a day) of 36 mg/deciliter reported a 3-wk history of hearing music. Although she had bilateral hearing aids, no other cause for this form of tinnitus could be found. After reducing aspirin intake to 6 tablets a day, the music stopped; there has been no reoccurrence.

88. Hallam, R. S.; Jakes, Simon C.; Chambers, C.; Hinchcliffe, Ronald.
"A comparison of different methods for assessing the 'intensity' of tinnitus." *Acta Oto-Laryngologica* 99.5–6 (May–Jun1985): 501–508.

ABSTRACT: Investigated the effect of hearing threshold on loudness matches expressed in sensation level (SL) by 82 Subjects (aged 18–78 yrs) with tinnitus and different degrees of hearing loss (HL). The loudness match expressed in SL was found to be a function of threshold. Correlations were determined between psychological scales of tinnitus complaint (reported loudness, distress, intrusiveness, and others) and loudness match expressed in HL, SL, sones, or personal loudness units (PLUs). Only matches expressed in PLUs were significantly correlatd with reported loudness or other psychological scales. The PLU transformation, derived from an individually determined loudness function, produced values that were generally independent of other audiometric measures. It is therefore recommended for assessing tinnitus intensity.

89. Jakes, Simon C.; Hallam, Richard S.; Chambers, Christine; Hinchcliffe, Ronald.
"A factor analytical study of tinnitus complaint behaviour." *Audiology* 24.3 (May–Jun 1985): 195–206.

ABSTRACT: Conducted 2 factor analyses on various self–rated complaints about tinnitus and related neuro–otological symptoms, together with audiometric measurements of tinnitus intensity (masking level and loudness matching levels). Subjects were 82 patients (mean age 50.4 yrs) who attended a neuro–otology clinic and whose main presenting symptom was tinnitus. Two general tinnitus complaint factors were identified: intrusiveness of tinnitus and distress due to tinnitus. Three specific tinnitus complaint factors were also found: sleep disturbance, medication use, and interference with passive auditory entertainments. Other neuro–otological symptoms and the audiometric measures did not load on these factors. An exception was provided by loudness matches at 1 kHz, which had a small loading on the intrusiveness factor. Self–rated loudness had a high loading on this factor. Otherwise, loudness (either self–rated or determined by loudness matching) was unrelated to complaint dimensions. The clinical implications of the multifactorial nature of tinnitus complaint behavior are considered. (French abstract)

90. Maurizi, Maurizio, et al.
"Contribution to the differentiation of peripheral versus central tinnitus via auditory brain stem response evaluation." *Audiology* 24.3 (May–Jun 1985): 207–216.

ABSTRACT: Evaluated auditory brain–stem response (ABR) parameters in 54 23–78 yr olds with unilateral idiopathic subjective tinnitus to verify the possibility of detecting its site of origin. All Subjects had normal hearing or a symmetrical bilateral sensorineural hearing loss. Subjects, classified on the basis of their mean auditory threshold and masking curve, underwent a residual inhibition (RI) test and ipsilateral narrow–band noise making before a 2nd ABR test was performed. Subjects with positive RI made up the A+ group, while those with negative RI made up the A– group. Main characteristics observed were an increase of the mean latency values of wave I in the tinnitus ear in the A+ group, while the values of the affected and unaffected ears almost overlapped after masking. An increase in the latency values of wave V, unaffected by the masking procedure, was observed in A– Subjects. The occurrence of waves I and III was often affected in the tinnitus ears in both groups, but it increased after masking only in the A– Subjects. It is concluded that there may be a substantial difference concerning ABR parameters between the Subjects in whom residual tinnitus masking is demonstrable and those in whom it is not. (French abstract)

91. Ireland, Christine E.; Wilson, Peter H.; Tonkin, John P.; Platt-Hepworth, Sarah.
"An evaluation of relaxation training in the treatment of tinnitus." *Behaviour Research & Therapy* 23.4 (1985): 423–430.

ABSTRACT: Evaluated the effectiveness of progressive muscular relaxation training in the treatment of tinnitus in 30 28–76 yr old patients who received either relaxation training with counterdemand instructions, relaxation training with neutral demand instructions, or no treatment. Assessment of subjective tinnitus severity, sleep difficulties, depression, and anxiety was conducted at pretreatment, posttreatment, and 6–wk follow-up, using daily monitoring, a sleep diary, the Beck Depression Inventory (BDI), and the State-Trait Anxiety Inventory (State form). No significant effects for relaxation training were found on any measure. Only the BDI improved significantly from pre- to post-treatment, but the degree of change was equivalent for both treated and untreated groups. While this study suggests that relaxation training is not an effective treatment for tinnitus, a number of explanations for the findings are offered.

92. Hallam, R. S.; Jakes, Simon C.
"Tinnitus: Differential effects of therapy in a single case." *Behaviour Research & Therapy* 23.6 (1985): 691–694.

ABSTRACT: Presents the case of a 60–yr–old male with tinnitus to illustrate the differential effects of psychological therapy on the sensory and affective components of tinnitus. Results of 11 sessions of therapy and a 1–yr follow-up show that, although Subject's self–rated loudness remained relatively unchanged, his development of tolerance reduced the associated handicap. The present authors attribute this positive change to the successful modification (via psychological techniques such as relaxation and imagery) of the negative meanings Subject had attributed to tinnitus noises.

93. Gerber, Kenneth E.; Nehemkis, Alexis M.; Charter, Richard A.; Jones, Howard C.
"Is tinnitus a psychological disorder?" *International Journal of Psychiatry in Medicine* 15.1 (1985-86): 81–87.

ABSTRACT: Examined several personality correlates of subjective tinnitus in 45 male patients (28–84 yrs of age) referred to the audiology clinic of a large VA Medical Center with constant tinnitus of at least 6 mo duration. Information was also collected on etiology, onset and chronicity, medications, prior treatment and related medical problems. Four standard psychological tests (MMPI, 16 PF, Rotter's Internal–External Locus of Control Scale and Holmes and Rahe Life Stress Scale) were administered to Subjects, in addition to a comprehensive audiologic and otologic evaluation. The expected psychosomatic characteristics of this patient population did not emerge as had been predicted from previous reports in the literature. Findings suggest that tinnitus may have an unwarranted reputation as a psychopathological disorder. It is concluded that conventional psychotherapy is less effective than standard audiologic approaches to the treatment of tinnitus.

94. Hallam, R. S.; Stephens, S. D.
"Vestibular disorder and emotional distress." *Journal of Psychosomatic Research* 29.4 (1985): 407–413.

ABSTRACT: Administered the Crown–Crisp Experiential Index (CCEI) to 62 tinnitus sufferers (aged 20–78 yrs), some of whom also complained of dizziness, to examine whether the complaint of dizziness would be associated with higher scores on the anxiety scales of the CCEI. This hypothesis was confirmed. Subjects complaining of dizziness obtained much higher scores on Phobic and Somatic Anxiety scales in particular. However, the complaint of dizziness was completely uncorrelated with objective assessments of balance, and there was no effect of balance, objectively assessed, in moderating the association between the complaint of dizziness and anxiety. The results highlight the complex relationship between vestibular dysfunction and complaint behavior.

95. Scott, Berit; Lindberg, Per; Lyttkens, Leif; Melin, Lennart.
"Psychological treatment of tinnitus: An experimental group study."

Scandinavian Audiology 14.4 (1985): 223–230.

ABSTRACT: 22 32–72 yr old patients with moderately severe to severe subjective tinnitus were randomly assigned to a treatment group and waiting–list control group. Treatment was given with a coping technique and comprised 10 1–hr sessions. Following a corresponding period without treatment, the control group was treated similarly. Daily self–recording of the subjective tinnitus loudness, the discomfort from the tinnitus, depression, and irritation was performed before and after treatment. Psychoacoustic measurement was undertaken on 3 occasions. The treatment group improved significantly more than the waiting–list control group. After treatment of the latter group, combined data of both groups showed statistically significant improvements in all variables. Results show that tinnitus annoyance can be treated by psychological methods.

96. Duckro, Paul N.; Pollard, C. Alec; Bray, Hugh D.; Scheiter, Luci.
"Comprehensive behavioral management of complex tinnitus: A case illustration." *Biofeedback & Self Regulation* 9.4 (Dec 1984): 459–469.

ABSTRACT: Describes a program for behavioral management of complex tinnitus and reviews the clinical characteristics and typical treatment of the condition. Psychosocial sequelae are discussed in terms of their exacerbation of the symptom and their potential as foci of treatment. A case illustration is provided with a description of the treatment process. The program discussed by the present authors includes biofeedback therapy, pain management training, social skills training, assertion training, in vivo exposure to being alone, cognitive treatment of depression, and marital therapy.

97. Ince, Laurence P.; Greene, Renee Y.; Alba, Augusta; Zaretsky, Herbert H.
"Learned self–control of tinnitus through a matching–to–sample feedback technique: A clinical investigation." *Journal of Behavioral Medicine* 7.4 (Dec 1984): 355–365.

ABSTRACT: Reported 2 cases of a 36–yr–old male and a 36–yr–old female with subjective tinnitusaurium, who were treated successfully with a matching–to–sample procedure through which they were taught to reduce their tinnitus. Following baseline evaluations, Subjects' experienced tinnitus was reproduced audiometrically in terms of loudness, frequency, and quality. This was presented to them in the noninvolved ear and was gradually reduced within sessions. Subjects were required to concentrate on reducing their tinnitus until an equal match was achieved between it and the stimulus sound at each new decibel level. Both Subjects gained control over their tinnitus, reducing it markedly from baseline levels. This procedure is viewed as an advance over other techniques not only in that it significantly reduces the tinnitus, but in that it is achieved through the Subject's own control, providing psychological benefit.

98. Tyler, Richard S.; Conrad–Armes, David; Smith, Pauline A.
"Postmasking effects of sensorineural tinnitus: A preliminary investigation. *Journal of Speech & Hearing Research* 27.3 (Sep 1984): 466–474.

ABSTRACT: Measured the perception of tinnitus after the termination of a masker in 10 40–72 yr old Subjects with sensorineural tinnitus. Results show 5 patterns, not previously described, of tinnitus loudness after masker. For most Subjects tinnitus was present immediately after termination. At higher–levels and longer–durations, different patterns emerged for different Subjects: The tinnitus was (1) present immediately after the masker but at a softer loudness, (2) absent immediately after the masker but reappeared at softer loudness, (3) absent immediately after the masker but reappeared at premasker loudness, and (4) immediately present and louder than normal.

99. Lechtenberg, Richard; Shulman, Abraham.
"The neurologic implications of tinnitus." *Archives of Neurology* 41.7 (Jul 1984): 718–721.

ABSTRACT: 121 patients (aged 19–87 yrs) who presented with chronic tinnitus (a condition in which noise without an objectively verifiable source in the environment is perceived by the patient) received an otologic examination and a neurological evaluation that included a computed tomography. It was found that 21 percent of the Subjects had neurologic diseases that were the probable cause of the tinnitus, while 23 percent had related neurological problems. 52 percent had tinnitus of undetermined origin. It is noted that tinnitus may be the only symptom of a posterior fossa tumor or an early symptom of progressive degenerative neurologic disease.

100. Burns, Edward M.
"A comparison of variability among measurements of subjective tinnitus and objective stimuli." *Audiology* 23.4 (Jul–Aug 1984): 426–440.

ABSTRACT: Trained 8 patients with subjective tinnitus in pitch–matching, loudness–matching, and simultaneous–masking tasks using narrow–band noise and/or pure–tone stimuli. Three of the Subjects had normal audiometric thresholds and reported bilateral tinnitus (BT); 3 others had high–frequency sensorineural losses (HFSL) and reported BT. One Subject had a unilateral HFSL of unknown etiology with unilateral tinnitus (UT), and the last Subject had unilateral high–frequency loss associated with Meniere's disease and reported UT. Extensive pitch–matching, loudness–matching and masking measurements were obtained for the Subjects' tinnitus, after which the same measurements were obtained for objective stimuli that approximated the frequency and intensity of the tinnitus. No evidence of frequency–specific masking of tinnitus was seen in any of the Subjects, although such evidence was obtained for the masking of objective stimuli. Results suggest that the large variability in matches to tinnitus and the lack of normal frequency–specific masking of tinnitus in these Subjects may reflect interactions at levels higher than the end–organ rather than a degradation in peripheral auditory function. (French abstract)

101. Penner, M. J.
"Equal–loudness contours using subjective tinnitus as the standard. *Journal of Speech & Hearing Research* 27.2 (Jun 1984): 274–279.

ABSTRACT: Examined the level of comparison tones (Co) of various frequencies that were judged to be as loud as the tinnitus for 6 patients with sensorineural hearing loss and tinnitus caused by noise exposure. When the loudness of the tinnitus was assumed to be fixed at L sones, then the level, P, of the Co was nearly predicted from the equation $L = K (P - p -\text{sub–0})^{.6}$, where p –

sub–0 was the absolute threshold of the Co used for the match. The rate of increase of loudness depended on the threshold of the Co. For persons with high–frequency sensorineural hearing loss, therefore, the sensation level of the Co is always smaller in the region of loss than in the normal region. It follows that the sensation level of the Co does not reflect the loudness of the tinnitus.

102. Odkvist, L. M.; Bergholtz, L. M.; Lundgren, A.
"Topical Gentamycin treatment for disabling Meniere's disease." Transactions of the XXIIth Congress of the Scandinavian Oto-Laryngological Society: The vestibular system (1984). CONFERENCE PAPER *Acta Oto-Laryngologica* 412 (1984 Suppl): 74–76.

ABSTRACT: 16 patients (aged 40–62 yrs) who were seriously disabled by Meniere's disease (MD) and had been unresponsive to previous treatment attempts were treated with 3–11 local intratympanic administrations of gentamicin. Individual doses were approximately 0.5–1.0 ml. Results at 1–6 yr follow-up indicate that gentamicin was effective in eliminating vertigo in 14 Subjects who reported relief from tinnitus and feelings of unsteadiness and fullness in the ear. Gentamicin is recommended as a treatment alternative for MD; limitations of its use are noted

103. Banfai, P.; Hortmann, G.; Karczag, A.; Luers, Sr. Petra.
"Selection of patients. Proceedings of the Second International Symposium: Cochlear implants CONFERENCE PAPER (1983, Paris, France). Acta Oto-Laryngologica 411 (1984 Suppl): 147–156.

ABSTRACT: Reports results of the evaluation of 284 patients as candidates for cochlear implants. 46 12–60 yr old Subjects had cochlear implants. 43 Subjects were unsuitable because they had no residual hearing. In 7 Subjects, no hearing nerve function was detected, and 1 Subject had chronic otitis media. 20 children under 10 yrs old and 6 adults over 60 yrs of age were rejected. Seven Subjects were poorly motivated and 11 were diagnosed as having psychoneurosis; they were not implanted. Two Subjects had no reliable hearing training available at home; 12 Subjects were rejected because of low IQ. Implantation was rejected by 12 suitable Subjects because of the surgical procedure involved, while 13 suitable Subjects dropped out because their unrealistically high hopes of success were not met when the procedure was explained. 101 Subjects were listed for cochlear implantation. Age limits and implantation for pre-postlingual patients and those with tinnitus are discussed

104. Morgon, A. et al.
"Cochlear implant: Experience of the Lyon team." Proceedings of the Second International Symposium: Cochlear implants CONFERENCE PAPER (1983, Paris, France). *Acta Oto-Laryngologica* 411 (1984 Suppl): 195 –203.

ABSTRACT: Contends that an audiogram and a psychological examination (analyzing patient motivation) are necessary before cochlear implantation may be considered. It is suggested that the outside prosthesis and the implanted prosthesis must be miniaturized in the future to facilitate implants in deaf children. Future prostheses must also be used continuously, like any hearing aid. In a study of 211 2–18 yr old deaf children, only 3 cases (Subjects who had no oralization) were potential implant patients. During surgery, the electrophysiological response must be recorded. Clinical results for 2 males (aged 54 and 55 yrs) who received a cochlear prosthesis show improved lipreading scores, the disappearance of tinnitus, and changes in Subjects' affectivity and in their social demeanor.

105. Dowell, R. C.; Webb, R. L.; Clark, G. M.
"Clinical results using a multiple–channel cochlear prosthesis." Proceedings of the Second International Symposium: Cochlear implants CONFERENCE PAPER (1983, Paris, France). *Acta Oto-Laryngologica* 411 (1984 Suppl): 230–236.

ABSTRACT: Evaluated the progress of 8 22–67 yr old profoundly deaf patients who have been implanted with the Nucleus Limited multichannel cochlear prosthesis since it became available in 1982. All Subjects were everyday–occur for (at least) one signal frequency in the region without tinnitus. The frequency region of the tinnitus was inferred from pitch matches and from determination of the frequency region of the noise needed to mask it. For comparison, data from 3 normal undergraduates are included. For the Subjects with tinnitus, 2–tone forward masking patterns were decidedly different in the normal and the tinnitus regions. users of the device. Speech testing using the device alone showed consistently high scores for a variety of closed–set tests and significant levels of open–set speech understanding in most of the Subjects. Lipreading assessment with phoneme, word, sentence, and speech–tracking material showed significant improvement when using the prosthesis for all Subjects tested. Other benefits reported were recognition of environmental sounds, decreases in tinnitus, increased confidence in social and vocational situations, and improved voice control. One Subject was able to cope with interactive conversations over the telephone and 3 others were able to use the telephone in a limited way without special codes.

106. Lindberg, Per; Lyttkens, L.; Melin, L.; Scott, B.
"Tinnitus-incidence and handicap." *Scandinavian Audiology* 13.4 (1984): 287–291.

ABSTRACT: Surveyed 1,091 patients at a hearing center to assess the occurrence of tinnitus (TN). 59 percent claimed that they were troubled by TN. Stress symptoms such as headache, tension of facial muscles, and sleep disturbances were correlated to TN. A majority of Subjects with TN and hearing impairment regarded their TN as the major problem. It is suggested that efforts toward investigation and treatment of TN might considerably improve the prospects for hearing rehabilitation.

107. Lindberg, Per; Lyttkens, Leif; Melin, Lennart; Scott, Berit.
"The use of a coping–technique in the treatment of tinnitus." *Scandinavian Journal of Behaviour Therapy* 13.2 (1984): 117–121.

ABSTRACT: Investigated the effects of an applied relaxation technique combined with perceptual restructuring in a man in his late 50's suffering from tinnitus. In 9 1-hr sessions, Subject learned to use applied relaxation as a coping mechanism in situations where tinnitus was annoying, and he recorded tinnitus level and associated annoyance 4 times daily over 11 wks. Subject reported that the self control technique reduced annoyance during treatment and at 20 wk follow-up, suggesting that stress and anxiety related coping mechanisms may be successfully applied in the treatment of tinnitus.

108. Salvi, Richard J.; Ahroon, William A.
"Tinnitus and neural activity." *Journal of Speech & Hearing Research* 26.4 (Dec 1983): 629–632.

ABSTRACT: Measured the spontaneous discharge rates of auditory nerve fibers in a group of normal chinchillas and in 4 chinchillas with high–frequency, noise–induced hearing loss. In contrast to normal units, the high–frequency units in the noise–exposed Subjects tended to have elevated spontaneous discharge rates, high thresholds, and a lack of 2–tone inhibition. The change in spontaneous discharge rate across the distribution of nerve fibers is related to models of tinnitus and to human psychophysical data.

109. Cahani, M.; Paul, G.; Shahar, Anton.
"Tinnitus pitch and acoustic trauma." *Audiology* 22.4 (Jul–Aug 1983): 357–363.

ABSTRACT: 56 19–44 yr old males complaining of tinnitus were given an audiometric test and a test for identifying the analogous pitch of their tinnitus. All Subjects reported that they had been exposed to noise in the past. Subjects were divided into 2 groups on the basis of their audiometric test results: Subjects who showed a sensorineural hearing loss typical of acoustic trauma (Group P) and Subjects whose hearing was within normal limits (Group N). The pitch of the tinnitus in Group P was concentrated in the high–frequency range, whereas in Group N tinnitus pitch values were distributed over the low– and mid–audiometric frequency spectrum. It is concluded that different processes were involved in the generation of tinnitus in the 2 groups. Perhaps the cochlear damage that existed in Subjects suffering from acoustic trauma (Group P), which did not exist in Subjects with normal hearing (Group N), accounts for the different characteristics of the tinnitus in the 2 groups. (French abstract)

110. Dancer, Jesse E.; Conn, Marjorie.
"Effects of two procedural modifications of the frequency of false–alarm responses during pure–tone threshold determination." *Journal of Auditory Research* 23.3 (Jul 1983): 215–219.

ABSTRACT: Conducted 2 experiments with 20 normal–hearing young adults without tinnitus to determine whether auditory false alarms (FAs) are affected by the descending rather than ascending mode and by pulsed rather than continuous presentation of pure tones. Overall data indicate that FAs are significantly reduced during threshold–in–noise measurements by these 2 procedural changes. It is suggested that both changes act to increase stimulus certainty under difficult listening circumstances.

111. Hammeke, Thomas A.; McQuillen, Michael P.; Cohen, Bernard A.
"Musical hallucinations associated with acquired deafness." Journal of Neurology, *Neurosurgery & Psychiatry* 46.6 (Jun 1983): 570–572.

ABSTRACT: Presents case reports of a 75–y–old female and an 80–yr–old female with auditory hallucinations beginning after a long history of progressive bilateral hearing loss. The hallucinations included uniformed (tinnitus and irregular sounds of varying pitch and timbre) and formed (instrumental music, singing, and voices) components and were repetitive. They were affected by ambient noise levels; their content and speed were influenced by attentional and intentional factors. There was no evidence of global dementia or of epileptogenic or psychiatric disturbance. It is suggested that a combination of peripheral and associated central "disinhibition" may be responsible for such hallucinations.

112. Penner, M. J.
"Variability in matches to subjective tinnitus." *Journal of Speech & Hearing Research* 26.2 (Jun 1983): 263–267.

ABSTRACT: Studied the noise-induced sensorineural hearing loss in 3 tinnitus patients by matching a binaurally presented comparison tone to subjective tinnitus during a 20-day test period. As a control, results of matching an external comparison tone to a standard tone are also presented. The variability for tinnitus measurements was extremely large relative to comparable measures for objective stimuli. The relevance of this finding to the nature of tinnitus and to the construction of tinnitus maskers is discussed.

113. Wood, Keith A.; Webb, William L.; Orchik, Daniel J.; Shea, John J.
"Intractable tinnitus: Psychiatric aspects of treatment." *Psychosomatics* 24.6 (Jun 1983): 559–565.

ABSTRACT: 13 patients with chronic tinnitus (mean age 52 yrs) completed a form describing their medical, family, and social histories; the Eysenck Personality Questionnaire; the Beck Depression Inventory; and a leisure interests checklist. Subjects also completed an otologic assessment consisting of a case history, audiologic evaluation, and physical examination. While in a supine position, Subjects were administered lidocaine (100 mg, iv) and asked to report any change in the tinnitus and other sensations in the ear, and hearing was tested at once. Findings show that 11 Subjects reported a decrease in tinnitus; Subjects with a 51–100 percent reduction were assigned to Group A, while those with a 50 percent or less reduction were placed in Group B. The mean age of 61 yrs in Group A was 17 yrs older than the mean age of 44 yrs in Group B. There were 5 females in Group A and 3 in Group B. Group B rated higher on extraversion than did Group A, and Group A showed slightly more emotional instability than Group B. The more successfully treated Group A reported more depressive symptoms and leisure interests that Group B. Results suggest that there are psychological and social factors in the responsiveness of tinnitus patients to drug treatment.

114. Tyler, Richard S.; Baker, Lesley J.
"Difficulties experienced by tinnitus sufferers." Journal of Speech & Hearing Disorders 48:2 (May 1983): 150–154.

ABSTRACT: 72 27–88 yr old members of a tinnitus self-help group listed the difficulties that they had as a result of their tinnitus. Tinnitus was associated with hearing difficulties in 53 percent, effects on lifestyle in 93 percent, effects on general health in 56 percent, and emotional difficulties in 70 percent of the sample. Getting to sleep was the most frequently mentioned difficulty, and many

Subjects indicated that they experienced depression, annoyance, and insecurity. Clinical applications of the questionnaire used in the study are discussed.

115. Brattberg, Gunilla.
"An alternative method of treating tinnitus: Relaxation-hypnotherapy primarily through the home use of a recorded audio cassette. *International Journal of Clinical & Experimental Hypnosis* 31.2 (1983): 90–97.

ABSTRACT: 32 15–71 yr old patients suffering from tinnitus were treated with hypnosis. Treatment consisted of a 1–hr consultation with the physician, followed by 4 wks of daily home practice while listening to an audiotape recording of approximately 15 min duration. 22 of the Subjects treated learned in 1 mo to disregard the disturbing noise, a considerable gain in the ratio of therapy to time required. (German, French & Spanish abstracts)

116. Nicolau, A.
"Practici empirice "pentru aflarea si tamaduirea boalelor mintii" in trecutul medicinii romanesti. [Empirical practices for the diagnosis and treatment of mental disease in the past of Romanian medicine.] *Revista de Medicina Interna, Neurologie, Psihiatrie, Neurochirurgie, Dermato-Venerologie* 28.2 (Apr–Jun 1983): 153–160. Language: Romanian.

ABSTRACT: Abstract: Compares past and present practices of diagnosing and treating mental and physical illnesses. Descriptions are cited from 17th- and 18-century medical textbooks. Symptoms and treatment of melancholia, hypochondria, chronic intoxication, tinnitus, epilepsy, inflammations, and insanity are discussed. The medicinal use of alcohol and precious gems is considered. Dementia, delirium, confusion, and hallucination are defined.

117. Chiodo, June; Walley, Page B.; Jenkins, Jack O.
"A modified progressive relaxation training program in the rehabilitation of a hearing-impaired client." *International Journal of Behavioral Geriatrics* 2.1 (1983 Spring): 43–46.

ABSTRACT: Abstract: Describes the procedures used to teach relaxation skills to a 55–yr-old hearing–impaired female with a history of tinnitus. The standard verbal presentation of instructions was modified to include printed instructions, modeling, tactile shaping, and visual/verbal/tactile feedback. Subject was taught relaxation skills successfully, resulting in self–reported generalization to the home setting and concomitant decreases in tinnitus and time necessary to get to sleep. Results are discussed in terms of applicability to geriatric populations.

118. Tyler, Richard S.; Conrad-Armes, David.
"The determination of tinnitus loudness considering the effects of recruitment. *Journal of Speech & Hearing Research* 26.1 (Mar 1983): 59–72.

ABSTRACT: 16 Subjects with sensorineural tinnitus adjusted the level of a pure tone and broadband noise so that it was at threshold, equal in loudness to the tinnitus, and uncomfortably loud. Formulae to predict masking in loudness in tones, recruitment, and uncomfortable levels are presented; they present tinnitus loudness on an absolute scale. It is suggested that some form of central masking effect is operative in tinnitus and that tinnitus localized in one ear might have a retrocochlear locus.

119. Penner, M. J.
"The annoyance of tinnitus and the noise required to mask it." *Journal of Speech & Hearing Research* 26.1 (Mar 1983): 73–76.

ABSTRACT: Tested 11 sensorineural hearing loss patients to determine the intensity of broadband noise required to mask tinnitus. Findings show a significant correlation between the rate of change in noise that is needed over time to mask tinnitus (increases of up to 41 db over a 30–min period) and the reported annoyance of tinnitus as measured on a 5-point rating scale.

120. Mitchell, Curtin.
"The masking of tinnitus with pure tones." *Audiology* 22.1 (Jan–Feb 1983): 73–87.

ABSTRACT: Studied the tinnitus of 32 adults. The tinnitus in each Subject was matched to tones and bands of noise. Tones were then used to determine masking curves. Four types of masking curves were found, similar to those previously reported. Findings support previous studies where tinnitus masking curves were found to differ significantly from conventional masking curves. Audiometric curves were grouped according to severity of hearing loss to determine whether Subjects with similar threshold curves had similar masking curves. Similarities were noted in only 1 group: those with the least hearing loss. The relation masking curves and the success of masking therapy is discussed. (French abstract)

121. Spitzer, J. B.; Goldstein, B. A.; Salzbrenner, L. G.; Mueller, G.
"Effect of tinnitus masker noise on speech discrimination in quiet and two noise backgrounds. *Scandinavian Audiology* 12.3 (1983): 197–200.

ABSTRACT: Examined the effects of tinnitus masker noise on speech intelligibility using 20 Subjects (mean age 24 yrs) with normal hearing. Subjects listened to NU–6 word lists presented in sound field in quiet white noise and in cocktail party noise backgrounds with and without a tinnitus masker. Findings show little impairment while wearing the masker in quiet; substantial discrimination loss was observed in the 2 noise backgrounds. It is concluded that since conversational situations are generally noise–loaded, the masking noise delivered by the device may hamper the tinnitus sufferer's ability to communicate effectively. Effects such as upward spread of masking and temporal masking that are known to adversely affect speech discrimination in hearing aid wearers may be operant while using a masking device.

122. Becht, Adeline C.
"The effectiveness of deep muscle relaxation with positive imagery and cognitive meditative therapy in treatment of stress resulting from subjective continuous tinnitus in hearing adults. DISSERTATION. *Dissertation Abstracts International* 43.6–B (1982): 1968.

1. Hartman, Bernard–Thomas.
"An exploratory study of the effects of disco music on the auditory and vestibular

systems. *Journal of Auditory Research* 22.4 (Oct 1982): 271–274.

ABSTRACT: Examined the records of 575 university students given audiometry and queried on their attendance at discos and on certain symptoms (vertigo, tinnitus, headache, nausea, otalgia) often associated with the Tullio effect. 365 Subjects had attended discos; 128 had binaural >= 25 db hearing threshold levels at 4 and/or 6 kilocycles/sec, 82 had Tullio symptoms, and 44 had both audiometric loss and Tullio symptoms. Data indicate that attendance at discos adversely affected both auditory and vestibular mechanisms in some Subjects124.

124. MacLeod-Morgan, Crisetta; Court, John; Roberts, Russell.
"Cognitive restructuring: A technique for the relief of chronic tinnitus."
Australian Journal of Clinical & Experimental Hypnosis 10.1 (May 1982): 27–33.

ABSTRACT: A combination of relaxation and imagery was used to teach an altered perception of their chronic tinnitus to 3 female clients (aged 36–60 yrs), for whom medical intervention had proven ineffective. The hum that had been troubling Subjects became a cue for relaxation and peace rather than a constant irritant.

125. Rudin, Donald O.
"The major psychoses and neuroses as omega–3 essential fatty acid deficiency syndrome: Substrate pellagra." *Biological Psychiatry* 16.9 (Sep 1981): 837–850.

ABSTRACT: Pellagra was once a major cause of 3 mental disorders–schizophreniform, manic–depressive–like, and phobic neurotic–plus drying dermatoses, autonomic neuropathies, tinnitus, and fatigue. In this study involving 12 mental patients (aged 22–58 yrs), all 3 corresponding present–day mental diseases were found to exhibit the same pellagraform physical disorders, but to ameliorate not so much with vitamins as with supplements of a trace omega–3 essential fatty acid (EFA). Since present–day refining and food selection patterns deplete the B vitamins and omega–3 EFA, the existence of therapeutically cross-reacting homologous catalyst and substrate deficiency forms of pellagra are postulated.

126. Borton, Thomas E.; Moore, Walter H.; Clark, Sandra R.
"Electromyographic feedback treatment for tinnitus aurium." *Journal of Speech & Hearing Disorders* 46.1 (Feb 1981): 39–45.

ABSTRACT: Investigated the relationship between behavioral severity ratings of tinnitus and EMG activity recorded at the frontalis muscle in a 60–yr–old female. Although auditory biofeedbackprocedures were effective in decreasing and increasing EMG activity at frontalis muscle sites, changes in EMG levels were not systematically related to behavioral severity ratings of either tinnitus or annoyance. Psychoacoustic judgments of tinnitus parameters were similarly unrelated to EMG levels. Psychological strategies were developed by Subject that apparently were associated with increases as well as decreases in EMG activity.

127. Man, A., and Naggan, L.
"Characteristics of tinnitus in acoustic trauma." *Audiology* 20.1 (Jan–Feb 1981):

72–78.

ABSTRACT: Several parameters of tinnitus were investigated in 102 Subjects suffering from acoustic trauma. These parameters were then compared to results of hearing tests and subjective complaints. The most effective masking of the tinnitus due to acoustic trauma was by pure tones. A significant association was found between the matched tinnitus level and its description by the patient. There was also an association between the severity of the acoustic trauma and the perceived loudness of the tinnitus. (French abstract)

128. Rosen, Jeanette K.
"Audiological and non-audiological correlates of acquired hearing impairment in an adult population." DISSERTATION. *Dissertation Abstracts International* 41.N7–B (Jan 1981): 2549.

129. Penner, M. J.; Brauth, Steven; Hood, Linda.
"The temporal course of the masking of tinnitus as a basis for inferring its origin." *Journal of Speech & Hearing Research* 24.2 (Jan 1981): 257–261.

ABSTRACT: Results from 20 Subjects suggest that excess neural activity is the physiological determinant of tinnitus and is generated in the brainstem postsynaptic to the 8th nerve.

130. Penner, M. J.
"Two-tone forward masking patterns and tinnitus." *Journal of Speech & Hearing Research* 23.4 (Dec 1980): 779–786.

ABSTRACT: Forward masking is the masking of a signal by a preceding masker. For normal observers, if 2 tones are employed as the forward masker, the addition of the 2nd tone (which increases the masker energy) may make the signal easier to hear. This decrease in the masking effect (or unmasking) has been interpreted as evidence for lateral suppression in hearing. For 5 Subjects with tinnitus, all of whom had a sensorineural loss caused by noise trauma or noise exposure, there was no unmasking for (at least) one signal frequency in the region of the tinnitus. However, unmasking did occur for (at least) one signal frequency in the region without tinnitus. The frequency region of the tinnitus was inferred from pitch matches and from determination of the frequency region of the noise needed to mask it. For comparison, data from 3 normal undergraduates are included. For the Subjects with tinnitus, 2–tone forward masking patterns were decidedly different in the normal and the tinnitus regions.

131. Till, James A., and Goldstein, Howard.
"Acquisition of a verb–subject–object miniature linguistic system by adults." *Journal of Speech & Hearing Research* 23.4 (Dec 1980): 787–801.

ABSTRACT: Forward masking is the masking of a signal by a preceding masker. For normal observers, if 2 tones are employed as the forward masker, the addition of the 2nd tone (which increases the masker energy) may make the signal easier to hear. This decrease in the masking effect (or unmasking) has been interpreted as evidence for lateral suppression in hearing. For 5 Subjects with tinnitus, all of whom had a sensorineural loss caused by noise trauma or noise exposure, there was no unmasking for (at least) one signal frequency in the region of the tinnitus. However, unmasking did

132. Formby, C.; Gjerdingen, D. B.
"Pure-tone masking of tinnitus." Audiology 19.6 (Nov–Dec 1980): 519–535.

ABSTRACT: Two experiments examined the frequency most closely associated with a continuous atonal tinnitus (T) reported by a listener (the 2nd author, aged 39) with a sloping sensorineural hearing loss in his left ear. The masking levels required to mask the T were consistent with those reported necessary to mask the equally loud pure tone. (French summary)

133. Tarnopolsky, Alex; Watkins, Gareth; Hand, David J.
"Aircraft noise and mental health: I. Prevalance of individual symptoms."
Psychological Medicine 10.4 (Nov 1980): 683–698.

ABSTRACT: Surveyed approximately 6,000 urban dwellers (16+ yrs of age) who resided in areas of different aircraft noise exposure. Since no differences were found in the prevalence of manifest psychiatric disorders, the frequency of 27 individual acute and chronic symptoms was investigated. Many acute symptoms showed an increase with noise, and this was particularly evident for waking at night, irritability, depression, difficulty in getting to sleep, swollen ankles, burns/cuts/minor accidents, and skin troubles. Two chronic symptoms—tinnitus and ear problems—were more common in low noise conditions. Results are controlled for the effects of age, sex, and other standard epidemiological variables. Irrespective of their association with noise, most symptoms (chronic and acute) were more frequent among Subjects who also reported high annoyance.

134. Singerman, Burt; Riedner, Erwin; Folstein, Marshal F.
"Emotional disturbance in hearing clinic patients." *British Journal of Psychiatry*
137 (Jul 1980): 58–62.

ABSTRACT: 156 outpatients (aged over 21 yrs) scheduled for hearing evaluation were screened for psychiatric morbidity using the General Health Questionnaire (GHQ–30). There was an association between objective hearing loss and elevated GHQ–30 score. An association was also found between the presence of tinnitus and vestibular symptoms and elevated GHQ–30 score

135. Goodwin, Patricia E.
"The loudness of tinnitus." DISSERTATION. *Dissertation Abstracts International*
40.1–B (Jul 1979):154.

136. Abstracts of the proceedings for the Second Annual Meeting of the American Association of Biofeedback Clinicians, (Nov 1978). *American Journal of Clinical Biofeedback* 1.2 (1978 Winter): 83–90.

ABSTRACT: Topics include the use of biofeedback to treat pain, sickle cell crisis, business stress, hypertension, hyperactive children, tinnitus, muscle spasticity, and headache.

137. Chapel, James L., and Husain, Arshad.
"The neuropsychiatric aspects of carbon monoxide poisoning." *Psychiatric Opinion* 15.3 (Mar 1978): 33–37.

ABSTRACT: Describes the neuropsychiatric picture of a family of 4 who were poisoned by carbon monoxide from a faulty muffler. Two of the surviving three appear to have overcome most of the major complications but still have tinnitus and "forgetfulness." The most seriously affected member, a 13–yr–old girl, is still seriously handicapped by a frontal (limbic) syndrome and a temporal lobe seizure disorder with associated interictal psychosis.

138. Lackner, James R.
"The auditory characteristics of tinnitus resulting from cerebral injury." *Experimental Neurology* 51.1 (Apr 1976): 54–67.

ABSTRACT: A study of 6 patients with tinnitus resulting from head injuries indicated that tinnitus of central origin seems to have the same auditory characteristics as external sounds normally generated; by contrast, tinnitus of peripheral origin does not participate in the same forms of binaural interaction. The different characteristics of these 2 forms of tinnitus are the basis for the conflicting claims in the literature about the auditory characteristics of tinnitus.

139. Maeda, Hisao.
"[Two cases of pentazocine dependence.]" *Kyushu Neuro-psychiatry* 21.3–4 (Dec 1975): 209–215. Language: Japanese.

ABSTRACT: The 1st patient was a 49–yr–old male medical staff member who had been taking pentazocine daily for 2 yrs with a maximum dosage of 900 mg. He had previously been dependent on morphine and cloxazolam and had been depressive for approximately 6 mo before admission. The 2nd case, a 39–yr–old medical staff member, had taken pentazocine daily for over 2-½ yrs with a maximum dosage of 500 mg, but had no history of drug dependence. After admission, dosage was gradually reduced to zero by the 9th day. Both cases showed withdrawal symptoms such as tinnitus, tremor of the legs, lethargy, anorexia, chills, yawning, rhinorrhea, sneezing, sweating, lacrimation, paresthesia of all 4 limbs, anxiety, irritability.

Index

The Tinnitus Reduction Program
(Now on CD!)

If you suffer from tinnitus or hyperacusis you can join the thousands of people from all around the world who have experienced tinnitus reduction or complete elimination by using this program.

Kevin has just released a six CD program based on the original audiotapes he made for himself to help wipe out his tinnitus.

The first two CD's include 2 ½ hours of the latest in tinnitus reduction information. Updated regularly, you will know what Kevin is telling his clients who suffer from tinnitus. 90 minute telephone consultations and single session visits to see Kevin are $250.00. The six CD program often has more than enough information for many sufferers to create and develop their own tinnitus reduction plan. (Please start here first before e-mailing for a telephone consultation!)

In addition to the first two CD's you will receive four more specially designed self hypnosis CD's. These CD's are instrumental in many people's tinnitus reduction. For a sampling of testimonials from people who now experience silence or near silence, visit http://www.kevinhogan.com/ . The self hypnosis CD's literally help retrain the brain to focus both internally and externally on images and sounds that are not tinnitus.

These CD's are designed to literally create new neural pathways in the brain that do not have tinnitus "on them." Their effectiveness has been proven and the testimonials speak for themselves.

Order *The Tinnitus Reduction Program* by sending a check or money order for $139.95 to

Network 3000 Publishing
3432 Denmark Ave. #108
Eagan, MN 55123

For immediate processing of your order simply go to http://www.store.kevinhogan.com/ and click on "Tinnitus" Your program will be shipped today. Or you can call 612.616.0732 and leave your mailing and credit card information on our secure voice mail system. Do NOT suffer needlessly another day.